Applied Nutrition
Cats, Dogs, Wild Animals and Birds

DV Reddy

BVSc, MVSc, PhD
Professor and Head
Department of Animal Nutrition
Rajiv Gandhi College of Veterinary and
Animal Sciences, Pondicherry

Oxford & IBH Publishing Co. Pvt. Ltd.
New Delhi
(A Unit of CBS Publishers & Distributors Pvt Ltd)

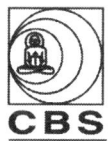

CBS

CBS Publishers & Distributors Pvt Ltd

New Delhi • Bengaluru • Chennai • Kochi • Kolkata • Mumbai
Bhopal • Bhubaneswar • Hyderabad • Jharkhand • Nagpur
Patna • Pune • Uttarakhand • Dhaka (Bangladesh)

Applied Nutrition

Cats, Dogs, Wild Animals and Birds

ISBN-13: 978-81-204-1774-8
ISBN-10: 81-204-1774-7

© 2014, Copyright Reserved

Reprint: 2019 2021

OXFORD & IBH

New Delhi
(A Unit of CBS Publishers & Distributors Pvt Ltd)

Published by Satish Kumar Jain and Produced by Varun Jain for
CBS Publishers & Distributors Pvt Ltd
4819/XI Prahlad Street, 24 Ansari Road, Daryaganj, New Delhi 110 002, India.

Ph: 23289259, 23266861, 23266867   Fax: 011-23243014   Website: www.cbspd.com
e-mail: delhi@cbspd.com;
cbspubs@airtelmail.in.

Corporate Office: 204 FIE, Industrial Area, Patparganj, Delhi 110 092, India
Ph: 4934 4934   Fax: 4934 4935   e-mail: publishing@cbspd.com;
publicity@cbspd.com

Branches

- Bengaluru: Seema House 2975, 17th Cross, K.R. Road, Banasankari 2nd Stage, Bengaluru 560 070, Karnataka
  Ph: +91-80-26771678/79   Fax: +91-80-26771680   e-mail: bangalore@cbspd.com
- Chennai: 7, Subbaraya Street, Shenoy Nagar, Chennai 600 030, Tamil Nadu
  Ph: +91-44-26260666, 26208620   Fax: +91-44-42032115   e-mail: chennai@cbspd.com
- Kochi: 42/1325, 1326, Power House Road, Opp KSEB Power House, Ernakulam 682 018, Kochi, Kerala
  Ph: +91-484-4059061-65   Fax: +91-484-4059065   e-mail: kochi@cbspd.com
- Kolkata: No. 6/B, Ground Floor, Rameswar Shaw Road, Kolkata-700014 (West Bengal), India
  Ph: +91-33-2289-1126, 2289-1127, 2289-1128   e-mail: kolkata@cbspd.com
- Mumbai: 83-C, Dr E Moses Road, Worli, Mumbai-400018, Maharashtra
  Ph: +91-22-24902340/41   Fax: +91-22-24902342   e-mail: mumbai@cbspd.com

Representatives

- Bhopal   0-8319310552
- Jharkhand   0-9811541605
- Pune   0-9623451994
- Dhaka (Bangladesh) 01912-003485
- Bhubaneswar   0-9911037372
- Nagpur   0-9021734563
- Uttarakhand   0-9716462459
- Hyderabad   0-9885175004
- Patna   0-9334159340

Printed at Chaman Enterprises, Daryaganj, New Delhi, India

Preface

Veterinary Council of India (Minimum Standards of Veterinary Education Degree Course - BVSc & AH) Syllabus and Regulations, 2008 came into effect from the Academic Year 2009-2010 onwards in all the Veterinary Colleges. The revised (first was in 1993) syllabus introduced certain composite courses to be taught jointly by the teachers of the respective departments. Two such courses are VMD-512 and VMD-513 that deal with Zoo/Wild animals and Pet animals & birds, respectively. My student-friends and colleague-teachers wanted me or rather prodded me to write on these new courses. The result is this present Textbook.

The textbook '**Applied Nutrition Cats, Dogs, Wild Animals and Birds**' consists of two sections (Part I and Part II). Pet Animal Nutrition (Cat and Dog Nutrition) is presented in Part I in five chapters (Chapters 1 to 5). Wild Animal Nutrition is presented in Part II in 14 chapters (Chapters 6 to 19). Important textbooks, textbook chapters, proceedings of the scientific conferences and research and review papers are given in the references. Composition of mammalian milks for eutherians and marsupials are furnished in the appendix.

Each section provides a structured approach to learning by covering all the topics in a uniform, systematic format. Some of the topics have been detailed beyond the syllabus level to enlarge the knowledge of the readers because of their importance in applied feeding. The topics are detailed in a straightforward and hopefully lucid manner. "Complete information in a comprehensible way" is the watchword of the book.

Though the textbook is termed as NUTRITION in continuation of my 'animal nutrition series', the book contains detailed information on taxonomy, control and conservation of wildlife, schedules of wildlife protection act, feeding management and feeding schedules of zoo/wild animals & feeding of common birds and pet birds. Information on feeding of sick animals -

therapeutic diets, metabolic diseases in wild mammals & birds and wildlife diseases is also furnished. Veterinarians are vulnerable to several zoonotic diseases. 'One Health Initiative' to attain optimal health for people, animals and environment and frameworks for vaccine-based interventions are mentioned.

The book is also useful to postgraduate students, teachers and scientists of Wildlife studies, Animal sciences and Veterinary sciences; zoo veterinarians, field veterinarians, personnel of Zoological parks, pet and wild animal lovers.

I appreciate the contribution of Dr. N. Elanchezhian for the balanced diet charts for dogs & cats and Dr. D. Sreekumar for information on taxonomy of the birds. I take this opportunity to express my gratitude to the publishers for their meticulous planning and intelligent publishing of the textbook. The services of Thiru B. Kumaran are appreciated for neat typing of manuscript. Above all, I thank God for His guidance and inspiration.

January 2014   **DUVVURU VENKA REDDY**

Contents

PART I

Pet Animal Nutrition

(Cat and Dog Nutrition)

PART II

Wild Animal Nutrition

PART I
Pet Animal Nutrition
(Cat and Dog Nutrition)

1

Digestion of Feed and Nutrient Digestibility in Cats and Dogs

General Information on Dog Breeds and Body Weights

Several breeds of dogs of variable mature body weights are reared as companion animals and to combat against rising crimes, bomb threats and drug trafficking. For example, the mature body weight of Chihuahua, 1 kg; Pomeranians, 2 kg; Great Danes, 50.0 kg; St. Bernard, 90 kg. The other breeds are German Shepherd/Alsatian, Labrador retriever, Cocker spaniel, Dobermann, Beagle, Boxer, Pointer, Poodle, Dachshund, Rajapalayam (Tamilnadu) etc. The birth weight is as follows: Pomeranian, 120 g; Beagle, 280g; German Shepherd, 400g; Great Dane, 450-550 g.

Dogs are Trained in Specialised Disciplines

Dogs are trained in specialised disciplines like tracking, explosive and narcotics sniffing, antismuggling operations and guard dog training. Trained dogs are deployed at various vulnerable places along the international border for preventing transborder crimes, as well as on VVIP duties, parliament security and at international airports. High pedigree dogs are reared. The Alsatians are multipurpose and are 'must' in infantry patrol. Police and Army maintain them for intelligence purposes. They are also good at sniffing out landmines and are trained to walk softly on suspected minefield. The Labrador retriever and the Cocker spaniel are good at sniffing and are used as guide dogs. The Cocker spaniels are preferred in sniffing operations inside aeroplanes and other cramped places. The Dobermann is useful in tracking operations. "Dogs are instruments which never fail the master".

Doberman are preferred: Police train German Shepherd, Labrador retriever and Doberman for tracking to detect crimes and for sniffing to unearth explosives and narcotics. Doberman were preferred by the Tamil Nadu Special Task Force to hunt sandal wood smugglers in the jungles. Doberman puppies after completion of basic training in obedience and discipline are used along with the handlers in hunting / search operations to catch the absconding persons. The Doberman pups are agile and could pick up scent and pursue clues vigorously. Ectoparasites such as ticks can be easily noticed on the Doberman and removed then and there while it is not possible in case of the German Shepherds (Alsatian) because of the amount of hair all over the body.

Differences between Dogs and Cats

1. Dog is an omnivorous animal while cat is an obligate carnivore.
2. Shape and arrangement of teeth: Dogs have more premolars and molars, with those in the rear designed for crushing, which is helpful in utilizing plant material. The upper P4 premolar (or carnassial) of the cat, when occluding with the lower molar, serves as a shear to cut animal flesh, and the cat does not have crushing molars.
3. Nutritional requirements: Cats have dietary requirements for certain nutrients that are found in animal tissues and rarely in plants. These include the EFA arachidonic acid, preformed vitamin A, and the aminosulphonic acid taurine. Dogs can synthesize these from nutrient precursors (linoleic acid, beta carotene and sulphur-containing amino acids) that are found in plants. Cats can synthesize only nutritionally insignificant amounts of nicotinic acid from tryptophan, although both nutrients are present in animal and plant tissues. Further evidence of carnivory can be seen in the high acivity of glucogenic enzymes in the tissues of the cat and the limited ability to conserve nitrogen, which would not be limiting in the meat diet with which cats evolved.
4. Cats are sensitive to a number of secondary compounds that occur in plants (e.g., benzoic acid) that can be detoxified by dogs.
5. In the cat and dog, salivary secretion has the special function of evaporative cooling and the parotid gland of dog secrets 10 times as the parotid gland in humans. Thus, regulation of body heat by this means is as effective as evaporation of sweat in humans.
6. Digestive tract morphology: Similarities and differences

Intestinal length: Dogs and cats have a relatively similar digestive tract except for its length. Intestinal length is one factor that influences the amount of time the food resides in the gut which in turn, influences the duration of digestion. Dogs with a body length of 0.75 m have an intestinal length averaging 4.5 m (small intestine = 3.9 m; large intestine = 0.6 m). Cats with a body length of 0.5 m have an intestinal length of approximately 2.1 m (small intestine = 1.7 m; large intestine = 0.4 m).

Absorptive surface area: The digestive tract of the dog or cat has a large absorptive surface area that serves to increase the rate of nutrient digestion and absorption as a result of the presence of villi. The surface area per centimetre of intestinal length is similar for the dog and the cat (jejunum, 54 and 50 cm^2; ileum, 38 and 36 cm^2, respectively) (Maskell and Johnson, 1993).

Gastric glands: A major difference in the gastrointestinal tracts of dogs and cats is the fact that the dog proximal stomach has a thinner mucous membrane with distinct gastric glands and the distal stomach has a thicker mucous membrane with less distinct glands.

Gastric mucosa: The gastric mucosa of the dog and cat stomach is divided into a narrow band of cardiac glandular mucosa and wide bands of proper gastric and pyloric glandular mucosa (Stevens and Hume, 1995). The cardiac and pyloric glandular regions secrete mucus and bicarbonate. The proper gastric glandular region secretes hydrochloric acid and pepsinogen. The feline gastric mucosa is uniform in comparison to that of the canine (Maskell and Johnson, 1993).

Caecum: Cat has a relatively smaller caecum than the dog, and a shorter intestine in proportion to body length, consistent with a carnivorous diet. In the dog, the caecum is a coiled appendage located distal to the ileocecal valve, while in the cat the caecum is not as coiled (Stevens and Hume, 1995).

Digestion of Feed

Ingestion, chewing, and swallowing are events consciously controlled by the individual. Thereafter, the digestive functions that begin in the back of the mouth with the initiation of swallowing are all reflex events (i.e., not under voluntary control). As food passes from the pharynx via the esophagus to the stomach, sphincters open and close under involuntary nervous control emanating subconsciously from the brain. All digestive secretions in the stomach and intestines are controlled by nervous and hormonal interactions as is the motility of the tract, which propels digesta in peristaltic waves towards the terminal end of the gut.

Digestion of feed involves a combination of mechanical, chemical, and microbial events, contributing to the sequential degradation of food components. Mastication and alimentary muscular contractions mechanically diminish the size of ingested food particles. Enzymes present in digestive fluids that are secreted into digesta in the stomach and small intestine instigate chemical degradation. Bacteria inhabiting the terminal section of the alimentary canal also produce enzymes capable of chemical digestion of those food components that have escaped hydrolytic digestion anterior in the tract.

Digestibility Studies in Cats and Dogs

Comparative studies have revealed a close relationship between intestinal characteristics, the natural feral diet, and nutrient requirements. Cats originate from a family comprised only of strict carnivores (Felidae), whereas dogs are omnivorous.

Total tract digestibility and ileal digestibility: Accurate quantification of the amount of nutrient consumed by the animal and that excreted in the stool is needed for calculation of nutrient digestibility. The difference between these two quantities, divided by the amount consumed, represents the quantity digested. This is an "apparent" rather than a "true" figure because some of the nutrients absorbed from the intestinal tract come back into the gut, and faeces contain a variable quantity of nutrients of nondietary origin (e.g., spent enzymes, pancreatic and gallbladder secretions, sloughed intestinal mucosal cells, bacteria). This is called total tract digestibility.

To quantify small intestinal digestibility, various methods involving surgical modification of the ileum have been used for both dogs and cats. Ileal contents may be collected before nutrients can be modified by large intestinal microbes. Ileal digestibility coefficients should be considered apparent rather than true values since endogenous secretions are part of the ileal chime. Attempts have been made to estimate endogenous secretions when animals have been deprived of feed for a time, when a nitrogen-free diet (or a low amount of a highly digestible protein [e.g., 5 percent casein]) is fed (for "true" protein and amino acid digestibility measurement), or when graded levels of a nutrient are fed with extrapolation to zero intake (Young et al., 1991).

Collection period: AAFCO (2003) protocols for dogs and cats recommend a 5-day diet adaptation phase followed by a 5-day period of faeces collection to ensure accurate digestibility measurements, although a 4-day collection period following a 3-day adaptation was found sufficient to measure apparent digestibilities in dogs (Nott et al. 1994). Cats exhibit more variable consumption and excretion patterns than do dogs. In the digestibility studies of cats, it is not unusual to have days in which consumption drops or when no stool is voided. Hence, this shorter period of collection was insufficient for accurate determination of digestibility.

Factors that Affect Nutrient Digestibility

1. **Plant factors:** Shields (1993) identified a number of factors that affect nutrient digestibility.
   - Ingredient sources and absolute nutrient concentrations can influence digestibility measurements.
   - Ingredient particle size reduction generally will improve digestibility, and therefore feed utilization. However, this reduces the quantity feed ground per unit time, in turn, leads to higher production costs, and reduced flowability of the feed.
   - Processing conditions in the preconditioning chamber, the pellet mill-extruder-retort process, or the drying oven could impact diet nutritive value.
   - Feeding management practices such as previous diet fed and amount of feed offered also could influence digestibility values.

2. **Animal factors:** Animal factors must be considered when evaluating digestibility. These include breed, age, gender, activity level, and physiological state.
   - Breed effect on digestibility was determined on 10 different canine breeds (Meyer et al., 1999) with varying body weights from 4.2 to 52.5 kg. The larger breeds tended to have higher faecal moisture content, less favourable faecal quality, and increased numbers of defecations. There were only small differences in apparent nutrient digestibilities among the breeds. The weight of the empty GI tract in small breeds is 6 to 7% of their body weight which decreases to 3 to 4% in large and giant breeds.
   - Effect of age and breed revealed that nutrient digestibilities were significantly higher in large dogs at all ages (11 to 60 weeks) studied, even though these (large) dogs had lower faecal scores and increased faecal moisture concentrations.
   - Age, too, is a factor impacting nutrient digestibility. In the study of Weber et al. (2003) it was observed that macronutrient digestibilities increased significantly with age (from 11 to 60 weeks) for all the four dog breeds (miniature dogs to Great Danes). It is not clear whether the lower digestibility values in puppies are due to higher feed consumption (relative to body weight or intestinal length) or due to their lower digestive efficiency.

- The limited information available on gender effects suggests that feed intake and faecal output are higher, and nutrient digestibility lower, for males of both species compared to females, with a suggestion that gender differences are greater for cats than for dogs (Shields, 1993).

3. **Environmental factors:** Housing and environmental factors could impact nutrient digestibility. Research with dogs housed in metabolism cages or covered kennel runs indicated that digestibility values were similar, regardless of housing system used (Shields, 1993). Temperature can exert its effect through either compensatory metabolic mechanisms to maintain body temperature or absolute amount of feed consumed.

2

Nutrient Requirements of Dogs and Cats

Dogs and cats are in the order Carnivora. However, feeding behaviour-wise, dogs are best described as omnivorous animals, while cats are true carnivores. The nutrient requirements of cat and dog vary throughout their life and are governed by factors such as age, level of activity, reproductive status, state of health and environmental conditions. The National Research Council (NRC), Association of American Feed Control Officials (AAFCO), the Canadian Veterinary Medical Association (CVMA), FEDIAF (Europe) and the Waltham Centre for Pet Nutrition (WCPN) have contributed greatly to the present day knowledge in the nutrient requirements of dogs and cats. FEDIAF represents the national pet food industry associations in the EU and from Bosnia-Herzegovina, Croatia, Norway, Russia, Serbia and Switzerland, representing in the region of 450 pet food factories across Europe. It has compiled the "Nutritional Guidelines for Complete and Complementary Pet Food for Cats and Dogs" in 2011.

Objective of Pet Animal Nutrition

The objective of pet animal nutrition is to promote its lifelong health as a companion animal to its owner, while economics of production matters in farm animal nutrition. Nutritional needs of pet animal are influenced by the animal's life stage as well as lifestyle. Life stages are growth, gestation, lactation and maintenance. Lifestyle of companion animals is quite variable: sedentary lifestyle of an apartment pet dog to active lifestyle of a house dog; dogs in street that have to hunt for a living are different; dogs used for work are very active.

Nutritional Requirements

Numerous factors affect the nutritional requirements of pets. These include age, breed, physiological growth status, sex, activity, health and reproduction.

Small breeds are often fussy, need highly palatable diet to be fed *ad libitum*, whereas medium, large and giant breed dogs are usually willing to consume less palatable diets and need to be fed in a portion-controlled manner. Small and medium breed dogs age slower, and need to be changed to senior diet at 9 years of age compared to 6 and 7.5 years, respectively, in case of giant and large breed dogs. Small breed dogs need a calorie dense diet because of a higher energy requirement per unit body weight as compared to larger breed dogs. Larger breed dogs are susceptible to high Ca intake and skeletal disorders due to rapid growth rate.

Expressing Requirements

Expressing a requirement relative to DM (Tables 7 and 13) or ME is the most convenient when formulating a diet, but expressing a requirement relative to metabolic body weight (Tables 4 and 9) may be more convenient when formulating a diet for an individual dog or cat. Unfortunately, requirements expressed relative to DM change with the energy density of the diet, and, in some instances, requirements expressed relative to ME may change with body weight.

Nutrient Requirements from NRC

NRC (2006) has used the latest scientific information to provide the requirements for individual nutrients and the scientific basis for the requirements of healthy dogs (*Canis familiaris*) and cats (*Felis Catus*) at several stages of growth and physiological states. This edition contains the latest data on requirements that are based on the utilization of nutrients in ingredients commonly produced and commercially available in dog and cat foods rather than only on purified diets. The Committee on Animal Nutrition recommended combining the data on dog and cat that was published separately earlier (National Research Council, 1985, 1986) because of overlapping use of feed ingredients, as a convenience to readers and for efficient presentation of the scientific basis for nutrient requirements.

NRC (2006) requirements are based on the following points. The energy density of the diet for both dogs and cats was assumed to be 4,000 kcal ME per kg. Requirements for growth of puppies are based on a 5.5-kg puppy that consumes 1,000 kcal ME per day. Requirements for adult dogs at maintenance are based on a 15-kg adult dog that consumes 1,000 kcal ME per day. Requirements of gestating and lactating dogs are based on a 22-kg bitch with eight puppies in peak lactation consuming 5,000 kcal ME per day.

Requirements for growth of kittens are based on an 800-g kitten that consumes 180 kcal ME per day, and those for an adult cat at maintenance are based on a 4-kg adult cat that consumes 250 kcal ME per day. Requirements of gestating and lactating cats are based on a 4-kg queen with four kittens in peak lactation consuming 540 kcal ME per day.

AAFCO Nutrient Profiles

AAFCO is an advisory body comprised of representatives from state, federal, and foreign regulatory agencies authorized to regulate the safety and labelling of animal feeds. A food that is formulated to meet AAFCO nutrient profiles must contain specified minimal and maximal levels of essential nutrients such as amino acids, vitamins, and minerals. Two minimal nutrient profiles exist for dogs and cats, one for adult maintenance and the other for growth and reproduction (gestation and lactation). Maximal allowed levels of some nutrients apply to both the maintenance and the growth-reproduction profiles. Thus, foods that meet the growth-reproduction profiles meet the maintenance profiles by default, hence qualifying for all "all life stages" designation. Levels stipulated in the AAFCO profiles were established largely by reliance on recommendations of National Research Council publications for these species. AAFCO profiles are similar to nutrient "allowances" rather than requirements.

Energy

The daily energy requirement is the sum of the energy that is required for resting metabolic rate, voluntary muscular activity, food-induced thermogenesis and maintenance of body temperature when the animal is exposed to adverse weather conditions. Energy is the most critical nutrient and hence is the first requirement to be met by the diet. Metabolizable energy is the preferred unit of energy for calculating the requirements in pets. Energy density is the principal factor that determines the quantity of food that an animal eats.

Since animals eat to satisfy their requirement for energy, all essential nutrients must be present in the correct amounts relative to the energy content of the diet. Energy itself is not a nutrient, since it is released by metabolism of macronutrients.

Fats and Fatty Acids

Dietary fats serve three nutritional functions. They provide a concentrated form of energy intake and are a source of essential fatty acids. They contain and act as carriers for the digestion and absorption of the fat-soluble vitamins. The level and type of fat in the diet can also make important contributions to its texture and palatability. Dogs have a high capacity to derive energy from fat oxidation and high fat diets proved to increase stamina and capacity for aerobic work in endurance dogs. Optimal performance in racing greyhounds, on the other hand, is achieved by feeding a diet with a moderate fat content.

Protein

Body proteins constantly being turned over, animal requires a continuous supply of amino acid building blocks. Dietary protein and amino acid requirements vary according to life stage and lifestyle; factors such as disease, environmental temperature and stress also affect them. Protein requirement increases in bitches during pregnancy and lactation. Protein requirements are also higher in working and racing dogs, reflecting the demands of increased muscle turnover and protein synthesis.

Energy Requirements of Dogs

Basal metabolic rate (BMR) is defined as the energy required to maintain homeostasis in an animal in a post-absorptive state (ideally after an overnight fast) that is lying down but awake in a thermoneutral environment to which it has been acclimatized (Blaxter, 1989). As an alternative, the resting fed metabolic rate (RFMR), is measured in animals that are not in a post-absorptive state, but otherwise meet the criteria for basal metabolism. Heat production increases when food is consumed. This dietary thermogenesis or thermic effect of food represents the difference between RFMR and BMR.

Basis for Establishing Energy Requirements

The mature body weights of dogs may range from 1 to 90 kg or more and, hence allometric considerations of metabolic body weight are of paramount importance. From a physiological viewpoint, energy requirements of animals with widely differing weights are not related directly to body weight but are more closely related to body weight raised to some power, W^b, where W equals weight in kilograms and b is an exponent calculated from the experimental data.

Brody et al (1934) equation: $70.5 \times W^{0.73}$

Kleiber et al (1961) equation: $70 \times W^{0.75}$

Heusner (1982) argued that the interspecies mass exponent in Kleiber's equation is a statistical artifact and suggested that the theoretical exponent should be 0.67 to predict the intraspecies relationship of energy to mass. This theoretical exponent describes the relationship between mass and body surface in bodies that are geometrically similar. However, dogs of varying breeds and body sizes are not geometrically similar (Kirkwood, 1985). For instance, with increasing size, dogs become relatively taller at the shoulder and relatively narrower at the hip. Hence, it is suggested that the interspecies mass exponent from Kleiber's equation (0.75) may be more suitable to describe the relation between mass and energy in dogs than the intraspecies mass exponent suggested by Heusner (1982). We will continue to use the $kg^{0.75}$, which is also recommended by NRC (2006). It is widely accepted and easy to calculate by cubing the body weight (BW) and then taking its square root twice.

Energy and Nutrient Requirements

Daily metabolizable energy and nutrient requirements for growth of puppies after weaning, for adult dogs, for bitches in late gestation and for lactating bitches are presented in Tables 1 to 7. These data are self-explanatory with footnotes and certain examples of calculations are also furnished for easy application. Data in Table 2 are given as minimal requirements (MR), adequate intake (AI), recommended allowance (RA) and safe upper limit (SUL) as an example of how NRC (2006) requirements for dogs and cats have been presented.

Minimal Requirements (MR), Adequate intake (AI), recommended allowance (RA) and safe upper limit (SUL)

Minimal requirement is defined as the minimal concentration or amount of a bioavailable nutrient that will support a defined physiological state. Adequate intake (AI) is defined as the concentration in the diet or amount of nutrient required by the animal that is presumed to sustain a given life stage when no minimal requirement has been demonstrated. The recommended allowance (RA) is based on the minimal requirement and may include a bioavailable factor. Where minimal requirement is not available, the RA is based on the AI. Safe upper limit, or the maximal concentration or amount of a nutrient that has not been associated with adverse effects, of certain nutrients is also presented.

Growth

Newborn puppies need about 25 kcal/100 g BW (Kienzle et al., 1985). Growing puppies require about two times as much energy per unit of body weight as adult dogs of the same breed (Arnold and Elvehjem, 1939). Later the requirement decreases to 1.6 times the maintenance (208 kcal ME/kg $W^{0.75}$) when the puppies attain 40% of the adult weight, and 1.4 times at 80% of the adult weight. The ME requirements of growth as given by NRC (2006) and FEDIAF (2011) are furnished in the following (See tables 1 and 2). The age at which a puppy will attain these proportions of adult weight will vary with the breed of the dog. In general, large breeds of dog mature more slowly than the small breeds. The rate of growth in the early stages being very rapid, most breeds of dog will attain 50% of their mature adult weight at around 5 to 6 months of age.

Table 1a. Daily metabolizable energy requirements for growth of puppies after weaning[a,b]

ME (kcal) = maintenance amount $\times$ 3.2 $\times$ [$e^{(-0.87p)}$ – 0.1]
ME (kcal) = 130 $\times$ $BW_a^{0.75}$ $\times$ 3.2 $\times$ [$e^{(-0.87p)}$ – 0.1]

Where: p = BW_a / BW_m; BW_a = actual body weight at time of evaluation (kg); BW_m = expected mature body weight (kg); e = base of natural log = 2.718

Example:
Labrador puppy 16 weeks of age, 17 kg actual body weight, expected mature weight 35 kg
ME (kcal) = 130 $\times$ $17^{0.75}$ $\times$ 3.2 x [$e^{(-0.87p \times 17/35)}$ – 0.1] = 1,934 kcal

a   This table refers to puppies after weaning.
b   Maintenance energy requirements of inactive puppies (such as pet puppies without opportunity and / or stimulus to exercise) may be lower by 10 to 20 percent, and maintenance energy requirements of very active puppies, such as Great Danes in kennels, may be higher; Source: Nutrient requirements of dogs and cats (NRC, 2006)

Table-1b. Average energy requirements during growth in dogs (Adapted from FEDIAF, 2011, p51)

Puppies*	Age	Energy requirement	
	Newborn puppies	25 kcal/100 g BW	105 kJ/100 g BW
Rapidly growing	Up to 50% of adult weight	210 kcal/kg$^{0.75}$	880 kJ/kg$^{0.75}$

| Actively growing | 50 to 80% of adult weight | 175 kcal/kg$^{0.75}$ | 730 kJ/kg$^{0.75}$ |
| Growing | 80 to 100% of adult weight | 140 kcal/kg$^{0.75}$ | 585 kJ/kg$^{0.75}$ |

* Overfeeding in puppies can result in skeletal deformities especially in large and giant breeds. Therefore, puppies should never be fed *ad libitum* and weight gain be closely monitored.

Table-2. Nutrient requirements for growth of puppies after weaning*

Nutrient	Minimal Requirement (MR)			Recommended Allowance (RA)			Safe Upper Limit		
	Amt./ kg DM ($\equiv$4,000 kcal)[a]	Amt./ 1,000 kcal ME[b]	Amt./ kg BW$^{0.75c}$	Amt./ kg DM ($\equiv$4,000 kcal)[a]	Amt./ 1,000 kcal ME[b]	Amt./ kg BW$^{0.75c}$	Amt./ kg DM ($\equiv$4,000 kcal)[a]	Amt./ 1,000 kcal ME[b]	Amt./ kg BW$^{0.75c}$
Growing puppies 4-14 weeks old									
Crude Protein (g)	180	45	12.5	225	56.3	15.7			
Amino Acids									
Arginine (g)[d]	6.3	1.58	0.44	7.9	1.98	0.55			
Histidine (g)	3.1	0.78	0.22	3.9	0.98	0.27			
Isoleucine (g)	5.2	1.30	0.36	6.5	1.63	0.45			
Methionine (g)	2.8	0.70	0.19	3.5	0.88	0.24			
Methionine & Cystine (g)	5.6	1.40	0.39	7.0	1.75	0.49			
Leucine (g)	10.3	2.58	0.72	12.9	3.22	0.90			
Lysine (g)	7.0	1.75	0.49	8.8	2.20	0.61	>20	>5.0	>1.39
Phenylalanine (g)	5.2	1.30	0.36	6.5	1.63	0.45			
Phenylalanine & Tyrosine (g)[e]	10.4	2.60	0.72	13.0	3.25	0.90			
Threonine (g)	6.5	1.63	0.45	8.1	2.03	0.56			
Tryptophan (g)	1.8	0.45	0.13	2.3	0.58	0.16			
Valine (g)	5.4	1.35	0.38	6.8	1.70	0.47			
Growing puppies 14 weeks and older									
Crude Protein (g)	140	35	9.7	175	43.8	12.2			
Amino Acids									
Arginine (g)[d]	5.3	1.33	0.37	6.6	1.65	0.46			
Histidine (g)	2.0	0.50	0.14	2.5	0.63	0.17			
Isoleucine (g)	4.0	1.00	0.28	5.0	1.25	0.35			
Methionine (g)	2.1	0.53	0.15	2.6	0.65	0.18			

Methionine & Cystine (g)	4.2	1.05	0.29	5.3	1.33	0.37			
Leucine (g)	6.5	1.63	0.45	8.2	2.05	0.57			
Lysine (g)	5.6	1.40	0.39	7.0	1.75	0.49	>20	>5.0	>1.39
Phenylalanine (g)	4.0	1.00	0.28	5.0	1.25	0.35			
Phenylalanine & Tyrosine (g)[e]	8.0	2.00	0.56	10.0	2.50	0.70			
Threonine (g)	5.0	1.25	0.35	6.3	1.58	0.44			
Tryptophan (g)	1.4	0.35	0.10	1.8	0.45	0.13			
Valine (g)	4.5	1.13	0.31	5.6	1.40	0.39			
Total Fat (g)				85	21.3	5.9	330[a]	82.5	23.0
Fatty Acids									
Linoleic Acid (g)				13	3.3	0.8	65[a]	16.3	4.5
α-Linolenic Acid (g)[f]				0.8	0.2	0.05			
Arachidonic Acid (g)				0.3	0.08	0.022			
Eicosapentaenoic & Docosahexa-enoic Acid(g)[g]				0.5	0.13	0.036	11[a]	2.8	0.77
Minerals									
Calcium (g)[h]	8.0	2.0	0.56	12[h]	3.0[h]	0.68[h]	18	4.5	1.25
Phosphorus (g)				10	2.5	0.68			
Magnesium (mg)				400	100	27.4			
Sodium (mg)				2,200	550	100			
Potassium (g)				4.4	1.1	0.30			
Chloride (mg)				2,900	720	200			
Iron (mg)[i]	72	18	5.0	88	22	6.1			
Copper (mg)[i]				11	2.7	0.76			
Zinc (mg)	40	10	2.7	100	25	6.84			
Manganese (mg)				5.6	1.4	0.38			
Selenium (μg)	210	52.5	13.7	350	87.5	25.1			
Iodine (μg)				880	220	61.0			
Vitamins									
Vitamin A (RE)[j]				1,515	379	105	15,000[j]	3,750[j]	1,044[j]
Cholecalciferol (μg)[k]				13.8	3.4	0.96	80	20	5.6
Vitamin E, (α-tocopherol) (mg)[l]				30	7.5	2.1			

Vitamin K			
(Menadione)			
(mg)[m]	1.64	0.41	0.11
Thiamin (mg)	1.38	0.34	0.096
Riboflavin (mg)	5.25	1.32	0.37
Pyridoxine (mg)	1.5	0.375	0.10
Niacin (mg)	17.0	4.25	1.18
Pantothenic			
Acid (mg)	15.0	3.75	1.04
Cobalamin (μg)	35	8.75	2.4
Folic Acid (μg)	270	68	18.8
Biotin[n]			
Choline (mg)	1,700	425	118

a   The values for Amt/kg DM have been calculated assuming a dietary energy density of 4,000 kcal ME/kg. (The term ≡ signifies equivalence) If the energy density of the diet is not 4,000 kcal ME/kg, then to calculate the Amt/kg DM for each nutrient, multiply the value for the nutrient in the column labeled Amt/kg DM by the energy density of the pet food (in kcal ME/kg) and divide by 4,000.

b   To calculate the amount to feed of each nutrient, multiply the value for Amt/ 1,000 kcal ME for each nutrient by the energy requirement for the puppy in kcal (calculated from Table 1) and divide by 1,000.

c   The values for Amt/BW$^{0.75}$ apply only to 5.5 kg puppies of expected mature body weight of 35 kg. To calculate the amount of a nutrient for puppies of different current or expected mature body weights, calculate the energy requirement from Table -1 and multiply this by the nutrient Amt/1,000 kcal and divide by 1,000.

d   For 4 to 14 week-old puppies, 0.01 g arginine should be added for every g of crude protein above 180 g and 225 g, for the MR and RA, respectively, of arginine. For puppies over 14 weeks of age, 0.01 g arginine should be added for every g of crude protein above 140 g and 175 g for the MR and RA of arginine, respectively.

e   The quantity of tyrosine required to maximize black hair colour may be about 1.5 - 2.0 times this quantity.

f   The requirement for α-linolenic acid varies depending upon linoleic acid content of the diet. The ratio of linoleic to α-linolenic acid should be between 2.6 and 16. Note that 0.8 g/kg DM value shown is the minimum RA of α-linolenic acid at 13 g linoleic acid per kg DM, resulting in a ratio of linoleic acid to α-linolenic acid of approximately 16.

g   Eicosapentaenoic acid should not exceed 60% of the total amount.

h   The RA for the calcium requirements of weaned puppies (of expected mature body weight>25 kg) for up to 14 weeks of life should not be less than 0.54 g calcium/kg body weight.

i   Some oxide forms of iron and copper should not be used because of low bioavailability.

j   For vitamin A, requirements are expressed as RE (retinol equivalents). One RE is equal to 1 g of all-trans retinol, and one IU of vitamin A is equal to 0.3 RE. Safe upper limit values are expressed as μg retinol.

k   1 μg cholecalciferol = 40 IU vitamin D3.

l   Higher concentrations of vitamin E are recommended for high PUFA diets. One international unit of vitamin E = 1 mg all-rac-α-tocopheryl acetate.

m   Dogs have a metabolic requirement, but a dietary requirement has not been demonstrated when natural diets are fed. Adequate vitamin K is probably synthesized by intestinal microbes. The vitamin K allowance is expressed in terms of the commercially used precursor menadione that requires alkylation to the active vitamin K.

n   For normal diets not containing raw egg white, adequate biotin is probably provided by microbial synthesis in the intestine. Diets containing antibiotics may need supplementation.

* Nutrient requirements of dogs and cats (NRC, 2006)

Adult Maintenance

The maintenance energy requirement (MER) is the energy required to support energy equilibrium, (where ME intake equals heat production), over a long period of time (Blaxter, 1989). The NRC (1974) suggested the equation 132 Kcal ME $\times$ BW$^{0.75}$ for calculating the maintenance energy requirements. Adipose tissue is metabolically less active than lean body mass. Therefore dogs with a smaller percentage of lean body mass (e.g. overweight dogs) have below-average energy requirements for their body weight. Ageing in dogs is associated with a decline in physical activity, which is associated with a decline in lean body mass and increase in fat tissue, and this indicates the reduction in ME requirements.

The ME requirements of adult dogs as given by NRC (2006; Table 3a) and FEDIAF (2011; Table 3b) are furnished in the following. The amount of energy a particular dog needs is significantly influenced by other factors such as activity, environment, breed, temperament, insulation characteristics of skin and hair coat, body condition or disease. When dogs are housed at an ambient temperature (which is below or over their specific thermoneutral zone) maintenance energy requirements increase or decrease by 2-5 kcal (8-21 kJ) per kg$^{0.75}$ for every degree centigrade.

The range of work performed by dogs may vary from the limited exercise characteristics of the apartment pet to the intense effort of the working sled dog (Table 3c). It is recommended to feed to thrifty body condition. A racing greyhound may require energy only 10 to 20% above that of maintenance. A sled dog working under polar conditions may require 2 to 4 times the maintenance requirements in order to avert significant weight loss. Working dogs in hot, humid environments may require 50 to 100 % more energy than similar dogs in less stressful circumstances.

Table 3a. Daily metabolizable energy requirements for adult dogs at maintenance*

Type	Kcal × kg BW$^{0.75}$
Average for laboratory kennel dogs or active pet dogs[a]	130
Above average requirements:	
Young adult laboratory dogs or young adult active pet dogs	140
Adult laboratory Great Danes or active pet Great Danes	200
Adult laboratory terriers or active pet terriers	180
Below average requirements:	
Inactive pet dogs[b]	95
Older laboratory dogs or older active pet dogs or laboratory Newfoundlands	105

a   Dogs kept in a domestic environment with strong stimulus and ample opportunity to exercise, such as dogs in multiple dog house-holds in the country or in a house with a large yard;

b   Dogs kept in a domestic environment with little stimulus and opportunity to exercise. Requirements of older or overweight dogs may still be overestimated; * Nutrient requirements of dogs and cats (NRC, 2006)

Table-3b. Practical recommendations for Maintenance energy requirements (MER) in dogs at different ages [Source: FEDIAF (2011), p50]

Age Years	Average	
	kcal ME/kg$^{0.75}$	kJ ME/kg$^{0.75}$
1 – 2	130	550
3 – 7	115	480
> 7 (senior dogs)	100	418
Obese prone adults	≤90	≤376
Breed specific differences :		
Great Danes	200	837
Newfoundlands	105	439

Table-3c. **Recommendations for Daily energy requirements (DER) of adult dogs in relation to activity**

Activity level	kcal ME/kg$^{0.75}$	kJ ME/kg$^{0.75}$
Low activity (< 1 h/day) (e.g. walking)	100	418
Moderate activity (1 – 3 h/day) (e.g. playing)	125	523
High activity (3 – 6 h/day) (working dogs, e.g. sheep dogs)	150 – 175	628 – 732
High activity under extreme conditions (racing sled dogs 168 km/d in extreme cold)	860 – 1240	3600-5190

Source: FEDIAF (2011), p50

Table-4. **Recommended Allowance (RA; g per kg metabolic body size) of growing puppies, adults and bitches in late gestation and peak lactation***

Nutrient	Growing puppies, Age 4-14 weeks	14 week and older	Adults	Late gestation & peak lactation
Crude protein, g	15.7	12.2	3.28	24.6[a]
Total fat, g	-----	5.9	1.8	10.5
Linoleic acid, g	-----	0.8	0.36	1.6
α-Linolenic acid, g	-----	0.05	0.014	0.10
Arachidonic acid, g	-----	0.022	----	-----
EPA & DHA, g	-----	0.036	0.03	0.06
Calcium, g	-----	0.68	0.13	0.82
Phosphorus, g	-----	0.68	0.10	0.58

* Adapted from Nutrient requirements of dogs and cats (NRC, 2006); [a] For small bitches suckling two puppies: 10 g/kgW$^{0.75}$; for medium-sized bitches suckling six puppies: 20 g/kgW$^{0.75}$; for large bitches suckling eight puppies: 25 g/kgW$^{0.75}$

Gestation

Weight increase (20 to 25 percent) in bitches during pregnancy occurs mainly after the 28th day of gestation. Considerable weight gain of foetuses occurs only after the 40th day of pregnancy. In addition, extrauterine tissue of the bitch may start increasing before the 40th day of pregnancy. Therefore, it is recommended that feeding extra energy for pregnancy start 4 weeks after mating. It may be 186 kcal ME per kg metabolic body size (Table 5).

Lactation

Energy requirements increase greatly and are influenced by size of the litter (Tables 6a and 6b). Bitches with large litters may require 3 or more times the maintenance energy requirement (460 kcal ME/kg $W^{0.75}$). Foods of high nutrient density are recommended for feeding at this time. Bitches suckle their puppies in general for at least 6 weeks. Offering food to puppies may be started at 2½ weeks of age at the earliest but should begin by week 4 of lactation at the latest. At that age, the quantity and nutrient content of the milk are no longer appropriate. It is possible to wean puppies at that stage of lactation, although this is not recommended as it may have undesirable effects on imprinting of puppies, which could induce behaviour problems later on (NRC, 2006).

Table-5. **Daily metabolizable energy requirements for bitches in late gestation (4 weeks after mating until parturition)[a]***

ME (kcal) = maintenance + 26 kcal × kg BW
Average maintenance requirements 130 kcal × kg $BW^{0.75}$
ME (kcal) = 130 kcal × kg $BW^{0.75}$ + 26 kcal × kg BW

Example: Body weight of bitch 22 kg
Maintenance requirements $22^{0.75}$ × 130 kcal = 10.16 × 130 = 1,320 kcal
Requirements for gestation 22 × 26 kcal = 572 kcal
Total requirements 1,320 kcal + 572 kcal = 1,892 kcal

a   For variations in maintenance requirements, see Table-3.
*Nutrient requirements of dogs and cats (NRC, 2006);

Table-6a. **Daily metabolizable energy requirements for lactating bitches based on number of puppies and weeks of lactation**

Requirements for lactation
ME (kcal) = maintenance + BW × (24n + 12m) × L
Extrapolated maintenance energy requirements during lactation: 145 kcal × $BW^{0.75}$
ME (kcal) = 145 kcal × $BW^{0.75}$ + BW × (24n + 12m) × L
Where:
BW = body weight of bitch (kg)
n = number of puppies between 1 and 4
m = number of puppies 5 and 8 (<5 puppies m = 0)
L = correction factor for stage of lactation: week 1, 0.75; week 2, 0.95; week 3, 1.1; and week 4, 1.2. *, **

Example:
Bitch 22kg, 6 puppies third week of lactation

Maintenance requirements = $22^{0.75} \times 145$ kcal = 10.16×145 kcal = 1,473 kcal
Number of puppies = 6; n = 4, m = 2; Stage of lactation-third week: L = 1.1
Requirements for lactation = $22 \times (24 \times 4 + 12 \times 2) \times 1.1$ kcal = 2,904 kcal
Total requirements 1,473 kcal + 2,904 kcal = 4,377 kcal

*   Expressed as a percentage of the mean daily milk yield during the first 4 weeks of lactation, milk production is as follows: 75 percent in week 1, 95 percent in week 2, 110 percent in week 3, and 120 percent in week 4.

**   From the nutrient content of bitch milk, the gross energy content is estimated to amount to about 1.45 kcal per g wet weight. The energy content of canine milk shows little variation except for the colostral period (Meyer et al., 1985b). Milk yield has been estimated to amount up to 8 percent of body weight (Ruesse, 1961; Oftedal, 1984; Meyer et al., 1985b; Scantlebury et al., 2000). These studies agree that peak lactation in the bitch occurs in the 4th week; * Nutrient requirements of dogs and cats (NRC, 2006)

Table-6b.   **Average energy requirements during reproduction in dogs***

Bitches	Reproduction phase	Energy requirement	
Gestation	first 4 weeks of gestation	132 kcal/kg BW$^{0.75}$	550 kJ/kg BW$^{0.75}$
	last 5 weeks of gestation	132 kcal/kg BW$^{0.75}$ + 26 kcal/kg BW	550 kJ/kg BW$^{0.75}$ + 110 kJ/kg BW
Lactation		**Kcal**	**kJoule**
	1 to 4 puppies	132 kcal /kg BW$^{0.75}$ + 24n × kg BW × L	550 kJ/kg BW$^{0.75}$ + 100n × kg BW × L
	Lactating bitch, 5 to 8 puppies	132 kcal /kg BW$^{0.75}$ + (96 + 12n) × kg BW × L	550 kJ/kg BW$^{0.75}$ + (400 + 50n) × kg BW × L

* Source: FEDIAF (2011), p51; n = number of puppies; L = 0.75 in week 1 of lactation; 0.95 in week 2; 1.1 in week 3 and 1.2 in week 4;

Table-7.   **Minimum Recommended Nutrient Levels for Dogs – amount per 100 g dry matter* Adapted from FEDIAF (2011), p14**

Nutrient	Adult	Early Growth (< 14 weeks) & Reproduction	Late Growth (≥14 weeks)	Maximum** (L) = legal (N) = nutritional
		Minimum Recommended		
Protein, g	18.0	25.0	20.0	-

Arginine, g	0.52	0.82	0.69	-
Histidine, g	0.23	0.39	0.25	-
Isoleucine, g	0.46	0.65	0.50	-
Leucine, g	0.82	1.29	0.80	-
Lysine, g	0.42	0.88	0.70	**Growth: 2.8 (N)**
Methionine, g	0.31	0.35	0.26	-
Methionine + cysteine, g	0.62	0.70	0.53	-
Phenylalanine, g	0.54	0.65	0.50	-
Phenylalanine + tyrosine, g	0.89	1.30	1.00	-
Threonine, g	0.52	0.81	0.64	-
Tryptophan, g	0.17	0.23	0.21	-
Valine, g	0.59	0.68	0.56	-
Fat, g	**5.5**	**8.50**	**8.50**	**-**
Linoleic acid (ω-6), g	1.32	1.30	1.30	Early growth: 6.50 (N)
Arachidonic acid (ω-6), mg	-	30.0	30.0	-
Alpha-linolenic acid (ω-3), g	-	0.08	0.08	-
EPA + DHA (ω-3), g	-	0.05	0.05	-

Minerals

Calcium, g	0.50	1.0	0.80a – 1.00[b]	Adult: 2.5 (N) Early growth: 1.6 (N) Late growth: 1.8 (N)
Phosphorus, g	0.40	0.90	0.70	Adult:1.60 (N)
Ca/P ratio	1/1–2/1	1/1–1.6/1	1/1–1.6/1[b] or 1:8/1[a]	-
Potassium, g	0.50	0.44	0.44	-
Sodium, g	0.10	0.22	0.22	Adult: 1.8 (N)
Chloride, g	0.15	0.33	0.33	Adult: 2.25 (N)
Magnesium, g	0.07	0.04	0.04	

Trace elements

Copper, mg	0.72	1.10	1.10	2.8 (L)
Iodine, mg	0.11	0.15	0.15	1.1 (L)

Iron, mg	3.60	8.80	8.80	142 (L)
Manganese, mg	0.58	0.56	0.56	17.0 (L)
Selenium, g	30.0	35.0	35.0	56.8 (L)
Zinc, mg	7.2	10.0	10.0	28.4 (L)
				Growth: 100(N)

Vitamins

Vitamin A, IU	500	500	500	40,000 (N)
Vitamin D, IU	50.0	55.2	50.0	227 (L) 320 (N)
Vitamin E, IU	3.60	5.00	5.00	-
Thiamine, mg	0.23	0.14	0.14	-
Riboflavin, mg	0.60	0.53	0.53	-
Pantothenic acid, mg	1.00	1.50	1.50	-
Vitamin B_6, mg	0.15	0.15	0.15	-
Vitamin B_{12}, µg	2.20	3.50	3.50	-
Niacin, mg	1.10	1.70	1.70	-
Folic acid, µg	18.0	27.0	27.0	-
Biotin, µg	-	-	-	-
Choline, mg	120	170	170	-
Vitamin K, µg	-	-	-	-

* Minimum recommended nutrient levels include a safety margin to prevent deficiencies due to animal variations and nutrient interactions;

** Maximum recommended nutrient levels on EU legal (L) limits or levels that are considered nutritionally safe (N) based on research data.

a For puppies of small and medium size breeds during the whole late growth phase (≥14 weeks);

b For puppies of large and giant breeds until the age of about 6 months. Only after 6 months, calcium can be reduced to 0.8% DM and the calcium-phosphorus ratio can be increased to 1.8/1.

Energy Requirements of Cats

Basis for Establishing Energy Requirements

The mature body weight of domestic cats (*Felis catus*) ranges from less than 2 to more than 7 kg. Mass exponents suggested for the calculation of metabolic body weight of domestic cats range from 0.4 to 1.0 (the latter exponent is used since weights of cats do not differ very much). Considering the findings of Nguyen et al. (2001) and the relatively uniform body shape of cats of different sizes, the cat might be a species for which the theoretical intraspecific allometric coefficient of 0.67 is justified.

For larger felids such as lions and tigers, it is unclear whether the intra- or interspecific mass exponent (0.67 or 0.75) should be used.

Energy and Nutrient Requirements

Daily metabolizable energy and nutrient requirements for growth of kittens after weaning, for adult cats, lactating queens and for queens in late gestation and lactating queens are presented in Tables 8 to 13. These data are self-explanatory with footnotes and certain examples of calculations are also furnished for easy application.

Table-8a. **Daily metabolizable energy requirements for growth of kittens after weaning***

ME (kcal) = maintenance amount $\times$ 6.7 $\times$ $[e^{(-0.189p)} - 0.66]$
ME (kcal) = 100 $\times$ $BW_a^{0.67}$ $\times$ 6.7 $\times$ $[e^{(-0.189p)} - 0.66]$

Where:
p = BW_a / BW_m; BW_a = actual body weight at time of evaluation (kg); BW_m = expected mature body weight (kg); e = base of natural log $\approx$ 2.718

Example: Kitten, 1 kg BW_a, 4 kg BW_m
ME (kcal) = 100 $\times$ $1^{0.67}$ $\times$ 6.732 $\times$ $[e^{(-0.189p \times 1/4)} - 0.66]$ = 198 kcal

* Nutrient requirements of dogs and cats (NRC, 2006)

Table-8b. **Average energy requirements during growth in cats**

Kittens	Age	Times MER
Rapidly growing	Up to 4 months	2.0 - 2.5
Actively growing	4 to 9 months	1.75 - 2.0
Growing	9 to 12 months	1.5

Source: Adapted from FEDIAF (2011), p52

Table-9. **Recommended Allowance (RA; g per kg metabolic body size) of growing kittens, adults and queens in late gestation and peak lactation***

Nutrient	Growing kittens	Adults	Late gestation	Peak lactation
Crude protein, g	11.8	4.96	7.40	16.10
Taurine, g	0.021	0.0099	0.018	0.018
Total fat, g	4.7	2.2	–	4.8

Linoleic acid, g	0.29	0.014	–	0.3
α-Linolenic acid, g	0.010	–	–	0.011
Arachidonic acid, g	0.001	0.0015	–	0.011
EPA & DHA, g	0.005	0.0025	–	0.0044
Calcium, g	0.410	0.071	–	0.565
Phosphorus, g	0.372	0.063	–	0.411

* Adapted from Nutrient requirements of dogs and cats (NRC, 2006)

Adult Maintenance

The equation of 100 kcal (418 kJ) ME per $kg^{0.67}$ proposed by NRC 2006 corresponds with a daily energy intake of about 60-70 kcal (250-290 KJ) ME per kg body weight(Table 10). The NRC specifies that this equation is only valid for cats with a lean body condition. However, many lean cats may need less energy (Riond et al., 2003, Wichert et al., 2007). Therefore it is justified to recommend a range that starts at 80 kcal (335 kJ) ME per $kg^{0.67}$ [about 50-60 kcal (210-250 kJ) ME per kg body weight] [FEDIAF (Europe), 2011]. Particularly for neutered cats and cats living indoors energy requirements may be substantially lower. In contrast to dogs, ME requirements appear to remain constant throughout life in adult cats.

Table-10.   Average daily energy requirements of adult cats*

Gender / Age	kcal ME /$kg^{0.67}$	kcal ME/kg BW	kJ ME /$kg^{0.67}$	kJ ME/kg BW
Intact male & female	80	50-60	335	210-250
Neutered and indoor cats	52-87	35-55	215-365	145-230
Active cats	100	60-70	418	250-290

Source: FEDIAF (2011), p52

Gestation

The pattern of weight changes during gestation and lactation appears to differ considerably between bitches and queens. Queens tend to lose body weight during lactation regardless of their diet (Scott, 1968; Hendriks and Wamberg, 2000). For satisfactory reproductive performance, body weight gain in pregnancy should include net tissue accretion in preparation for lactation, rather than gain only in foetal, placental, and associated tissue weight. Feeding for a 40 to 50 percent weight increase during pregnancy is recommended (Table 11).

Lactation

Queens suckle their kittens in general for 7-9 weeks, depending on litter size. Additional feeding of kittens may be started at 2½ weeks of age at the earliest and should begin during week 4 of lactation at the latest. At that age, the quantity and nutrient content of the milk are no longer sufficient for normal development (Hendriks and Wamberg, 2000). Milk yield increased after parturition until the 3rd or 4th week of lactation and decreased again thereafter (Table 12).

Table-11. Average energy requirements during reproduction in cats*

Queens		Reproduction phase	
Gestation		140 kcal/kg$^{0.67}$ BW	585 kJ/kg$^{0.67}$ BW
Lactation	< 3 kittens	100 kcal/kg$^{0.67}$ + 18 × kg BW × L	418 kJ/kg$^{0.67}$ + 75 × kg BW × L
	3 – 4 kittens	100 kcal/kg$^{0.67}$ + 60 × kg BW × L	418 kJ/kg$^{0.67}$ + 250 × kg BW × L
	> 4 kittens	100 kcal/kg$^{0.67}$ + 70 × kg BW × L	418 kJ/kg$^{0.67}$ + 293 × kg BW × L

L = 0.9 in weeks 1–2 of lactation; 1.2 in weeks 3-4; 1.1 in week 5; 1 in week 6; and 0.8 in week 7
* Source: FEDIAF (2011), p52

Table -12. Daily Metabolizable Energy Requirements for Lactating Queens*

Kittens	Energy Requirement
<3	ME kcal = maintenance + 18 × BW × L
	ME kcal = 100 × BW$^{0.67}$ + 18 × BW × L
3–4	ME kcal = maintenance + 60 × BW × L
	ME kcal = 100 x BW$^{0.67}$ + 60 × BW × L
>4	ME kcal = maintenance + 70 × BW × L
	ME kcal = 100 × BW$^{0.67}$ + 70 × BW × L

L = factor for stage of lactation from week 1 to week 7: 0.9, 0.9, 1.2, 1.2, 1.1, 1.0, 0.8

Example:
Queen, 3.5 kg BW at mating, 4 kittens, peak lactation (week 3)
ME kcal = 100 × 3.5$^{0.67}$ + (60 × 3.5 × 1.2) = 231 + 252 = 483 kcal

* Nutrient requirements of dogs and cats (NRC, 2006)

Table-13. Minimum Recommended Nutrient Levels for Cats -amount per 100 g dry matter* Adapted from FEDIAF (2011), p17

Nutrient	Adult	Growth and / Reproduction	Maximum** (L) = legal
		Minimum Recommended	(N) = nutritional
Protein, g	**25.0**	**28.0 / 30.0**	
Arginine, g	1.00	1.07/1.11	Growth 3.5 (N)
Histidine, g	0.30	0.33	
Isoleucine, g	0.49	0.54	
Leucine, g	1.17	1.28	
Lysine, g	0.34	0.85	
Methionine, g	0.17	0.44	Growth 1.3 (N)
Methionine + cysteine, g	0.34	0.88	
Phenylalanine, g	0.46	0.50	
Phenylalanine + tyrosine, g	1.76	1.91	
Threonine, g	0.60	0.65	
Tryptophan, g	0.15	0.16	Growth 1.7 (N)
Valine, g	0.59	0.64	
Taurine (canned pet food), g	0.20	0.25	
Taurine (dry pet food), g	0.10	0.10	
Fat, g	**9.0**	**9.0**	
Linoleic acid (ω-6), g	0.50	0.55	
Arachidonic acid (ω-6), mg	6.00	20.0	
Alpha-linolenic acid (ω-3), g	-	0.02	
EPA + DHA (ω-3), g	-	0.01	
Minerals			
Calcium, g	0.59	1.00	
Phosphorus, g	0.50	0.84	
Ca/P ratio	1/1 – 2/1	1/1 – 1.5/1	
Potassium, g	0.60	0.60	
Sodium, g	0.08	0.16	1.8 (N)
Chloride, g	0.11	0.24	
Magnesium, g	0.04	0.05	
Trace elements			
Copper, mg	0.50	1.00	2.8 (L)
Iodine, mg	0.05	0.18	1.1 (L)
Iron, mg	8.00	8.00	142 (L)
Manganese, mg	0.50	1.00	17.0 (L)
Selenium, g	30.0	30.0	56.8 (L)

Zinc, mg	7.50	7.50	28.4 (L) Adult: 60.0 (N)
Vitamins			
Vitamin A, IU	333	900	Adult & ᵧrowth 40,000 (N) Reproduction 33,333(N)
Vitamin D, IU	25.0	75.0	227 (L) 3,000 (N)
Vitamin E, IU	3.80	3.80	
Thiamine, mg	0.56	0.55	
Riboflavin, mg	0.40	0.40	
Pantothenic acid, mg	0.58	0.57	
Vitamin B_6, mg	0.25	0.40	
Vitamin B_{12}, µg	2.25	2.00	
Niacin, mg	4.00	4.00	
Folic acid, µg	80.0	80.0	
Biotin, µg	7.50	7.00	
Choline, mg	240	240	
Vitamin K, µg	10.0	10.0	

*   Minimum recommended nutrient levels include a safety margin to prevent deficiencies due to animal variations and nutrient interactions;

**   Maximum recommended nutrient levels on EU legal (L) limits or levels that are considered nutritionally safe (N) based on research data.

3

Nutrients and their Needs for Dogs and Cats

Carbohydrates in Dog and Cat Diet Formulations

The carbohydrate groups, enlisted from a functional perspective, are (1) absorbable (monosaccharides), (2) digestible (disaccharides, certain oligosaccharides, and non-structural polysaccharides, (NSP)), (3) fermentable (lactose, certain oligosaccharides, dietary fibre and resistant starch), and (4) nonfermentable (certain dietary fibre).

Essentiality of Carbohydrates

Carbohydrate is physiologically essential to the dog and cat. However, it is not essential in the diet of either species (except for the lactating bitch) provided that the protein level is high enough to supply sufficient gluconeogenic amino acids (alanine) and lactate to allow the maintenance of plasma glucose (70- 120 mg/dl). Research data indicated that, although pregnant and lactating bitches do not require a dietary source of carbohydrate, they have increased protein requirements when fed a carbohydrate-free diet. Feeding such diet resulted in a smaller litter size in beagles. Bitches fed a carbohydrate-free diet exhibited ketosis, which is associated with hypoglycemia. It was concluded that pregnant bitches require dietary carbohydrates for optimal reproductive performance and survivability of puppies.

Notwithstanding this, carbohydrates are a useful source of dietary energy, and cooked starch is generally readily digested by dogs and cats. Cooking is necessary to break down starch granules. The dog in particular is well able to digest starch, although quantities greater than approximately 65% of the total diet should be avoided.

Dogs: It is acceptable for carbohydrate to provide 40-50% of the total energy in the diet.

Cat: Carbohydrate should preferably be limited to no more than 30% of dietary energy.

Lactose Intolerance

The ability to digest lactose depends on the level of activity of β-galactosidase in the intestine. The activity of the enzyme is known to be higher in kittens. Lactose intolerance (characterized by diarrhoea) may be seen in animals suddenly given amounts of lactose beyond their digestive capabilities. Although individual variations in tolerance must be expected, digestive disorders have been reported in adult dogs with intakes greater than 0.6-1 g lactose/kg body weight/day. This is equivalent to about 10-20 ml of milk per kg B.W. daily. (The lactose content of bitch milk and queen milk are 3.7 and 4.9% respectively).

Though lactose is digestible, under certain conditions, its absorption in the small intestine is reduced and unabsorbed lactose is readily fermented in the colon. For diets containing lactose and sucrose, higher water content has been observed in the chime of the small and large intestine, as well as in faeces due to their osmotic effects.

Optimum crude fibre in dry petfood: Typical crude fibre level range from 2.5-5% and can vary as high as 24% in some specialized therapeutic foods (e.g. constiption, coprophagia). Its concentration in some reduced calorie diets may be 9 to 10%. Levels below 2.5% would likely impede normal bowel function. The recommended levels of fibre in dog and cat foods for optimum nutrition vary between 3.5% and 6%.

Though crude fibre is defined as that portion of a diet which is not soluble in either hot alkali or acid, it is realistic to think fibre as either insoluble and relatively inert (e.g. cellulose) or soluble (e.g. pectins, ispaghula,and gums) in water. Foodstuffs such as oats and oat bran are high in soluble fibre whereas wheat and wheat bran are associated with insoluble fibre. Soluble fibre has greater capacity to absorb and serves as a source of metabolizable energy through the process of fermentation in the colon. Further the short chain fatty acid, butyric acid, is a key source of energy for colonic epithelium.

Commonly Used Plant Ingredients

Cereal and legume grains, their byproducts and other plant components have different starch content (Table 1) and are the main sources of monosaccharides in pet foods. Feeds low in starch generally contain more fibre or non-starch polysaccharides (NSP), whereas starch-rich foods generally contain less fibre. Glucose and fructose are the predominant free-occuring monosaccharides in dog and cat foods. In the absence of dietary glucose, dogs synthesize glucose from amino acids and glycerol by way of gluconeogenesis.

The fact that cats are in a constant state of gluconeogenesis implies that glucose is important for normal metabolism in the feline species. However, they do not appear to utilize carbohydrates as rapidly as do dogs.

Table-1. **Starch content of some common plant ingredients used in dog and cat diets**

Product	Starch Content (g/kg diet DM)
Barley	500–516
Oats	400
Sorghum	620–741
Maize	630–728
Rye	520
Wheat	580–621
Peas	410
Horse beans	350
Pearl barley product (2% crude fibre)	530
Pearl barley product (7.5% crude fibre)	350
Pearl barley product (10.5% crude fibre)	300
Hominy feed	370
Maize bran	260
Rice bran (<3% husks)	270
Rice bran (3-10% husks)	230
Rice	810
Wheat feed flour	500
Wheat middlings	220
Wheat bran	140
Wheat germ meal	280
Dried potatoes	650
Dried potato pulp	280
Corn gluten feed	190

Source: Nutrient requirements of dogs and cats (NRC, 2006); Page 54

The recommended carbohydrate content of diets depends on amount of food consumed, caloric density of the food, and energy requirement of the animal (Meyer and Kienzle, 1991). Cereal grains are carbohydrate-rich ingredients used in formulating cat and dog foods. These ingredients are included at different dietary concentrations depending on diet type.

Dietary Starch and Feline Urologic Syndrome

Tarttelin (1991) suggested that feeding too high a concentration of carbohydrate may induce feline urologic syndrome since any persistent increase in urine pH, such as that induced by ingestion of high carbohydrate concentrations, results in precipitation of magnesium ammonium phosphate crystals (struvite). These crystals may block the urethra and predispose the cat to dietary induced feline urologic syndrome (Tarttelin, 1991). There is no known optimal starch inclusion level for the cat diet.

The Safe Upper Limit (SUL) of Dietary Inclusion for Various Carbohydrates

For many carbohydrates sources, there exists sufficient data to establish a level of dietary inclusion at which no adverse effects are to be expected (Table-2). These values are only for adult animals at maintenance. Adverse effects taken into consideration included occurrence of loose stools, elevated faecal water content, frequent defecation, marked reduction of nutrient digestibility, poor diet acceptability or palatability, and disturbances in nutrient metabolism.

Table-2. Safe upper limits of selected carbohydrates for adult dog and cat maintenance diets (g/kg diet, DM basis)*

Item	Dogs	Cats
Glucose	ND	50-150
Sucrose	350	50-150
Lactose	100	50
Cooked corn starch	ND	240
Cooked corn flour	436[a]	ND
Cooked potato flour	504[a]	ND
Cooked rice flour	441[a]	ND
Cooked wheat flour	491[a]	ND
Raffinose/stachyose	50	50
Fructooligosaccharides	40[b]	7.5[a]
Inulin	70[a]	ND
Mannanoligosaccharides	5.9[a]	ND
Xylooligosaccharides	5[a]	ND
Transgalactooligosaccharides	5.9	ND
Cellulose	94[a]	100

Guar gum	34	ND
Pectin	34	ND
Beet pulp	75	ND
Wheat bran	128	100
Peanut hulls	67[a]	ND
Tomato pomace	87[a]	ND
Oat Fibre	75[a]	ND
Fibre blend[c]	83[a]	83

* Nutrient requirements of dogs and cats (NRC, 2006), page no 73; ND = no experimental data available;
a Higher levels not experimentally tested;
b When mixed with sugar beet fibre in a 4:1 ratio;
c Mixture of Solka Floc and gum Arabic in a 3:1 ratio

Role of Prebiotics / Functional Foods on Intestinal Health

Certain oligosaccharides (fermentable carbohydrates) can be classified as prebiotics. Prebiotics are nondigested food ingredients that beneficially affect the host by stimulating the growth and activity of one or a limited number of bacterial species (probiotics) already residing in the colon (Gibson and Roberfroid, 1995), and also are defined as functional foods (Van Loo et al., 1999). Dietary fibre is directly involved in maintaining gut health through provision of short chain fatty acids (SCFAs), maintaining a healthy gut microflora, and possibility even preventing diseases.

Most of the intestinal bacteria can be divided into species that exert detrimental effects (Staphylococci, clostridia, and veillonella) or species that benefit the host (bifidobacteria, lactobacilli, and eubacteria). Diarrhoea, infection, digesta putrefaction, and promotion of carcinogenesis are examples of pathogenic effects, while defense against pathogens, prevention of infection, and reduction of serum cholesterol are examples of beneficial effects of the intestinal bacteria.

Prebiotic oligosaccharides include fructooligosaccharides (FOS), mannanoligosaccharides (MOS), glucooligosaccharides, galactooligosaccharides, and xylooligosaccharides. In addition to improving colonic microbial populations, prebiotic oligosaccharides also may positively affect small intestinal bacteria.

Role of Fibre in Weight Management of Dogs and Cats

The incidence of obesity increases with age and is more frequent in neutered than intact animals (Sloth, 1992). In addition, cats are affected by obesity at an earlier age than are dogs (Scarlett et al., 1994). Both insoluble and soluble fibres have been used as a means of restricting energy intake for weight control in companion animal nutrition. Examples are sugar beet pulp, pectins. Beet pulp contains both insoluble and soluble fibre components in a desirable ratio (approximately 17 to 20 percentage units of soluble fibre; Fahey, 1995).

Fibre dilutes the caloric content of food and offers an attractive solution for preventing weight gain in dogs and cats. Powdered cellulose is commonly used as a noncaloric bulking agent in reduced-calorie foods (Ang and Miller, 1991).

Dietary fibre has been thought to encourage proper weight maintenance through regulation of appetite (Butterwick and Markwell, 1997; Jackson et al., 1997), simple mechanical interference and other physical effects, and complex hormonal interactions (Rossner, 1992) determined by the nature and type of fibre (Blundell and Burley, 1987). It was demonstrated that gastric distension was a physiologic satiety signal in dogs. High concentrations of fibre in weight reduction diets may allow the animal to achieve a sense of fullness without a high energy intake

Glycemic Response of Diet in Feeding Diabetic or Obese Dogs

Feeds resulting in a lower glycemic response would be beneficial for diabetic or obese dogs. Nguyen et al. (1998) concluded that the amount of starch consumed is the major determinant of the glycemic response of adult healthy dogs (See Table 1 for starch content of feeds). Postprandial hyperglycemia and insulin secretion depend on the ratio of amylose to amylopectin consumed.

Dogs consuming the rice diet exhibited the highest average blood glucose values as well as the highest blood insulin values. Diets containing sorghum resulted in the lowest blood glucose, while diets containing barley resulted in the lowest blood insulin. Diets containing maize or wheat resulted in intermediate blood glucose and insulin values. These data indicate that the source of starch influences the postprandial glucose and insulin responses in adult dogs.

Glycemic Response of Diet in Feeding Geriatric Dogs and Cats

Companion animal longevity is important to pet owners and diet is one of the factors that impact longevity. In the geriatric animal, a small amount of dietary fibre facilitates the desired caloric restriction and aids intestinal function (Markham and Holdking, 1989).

Dogs and cats become increasingly less able to regulate their blood sugar concentrations as they age, and this disrupted carbohydrate metabolism at times leads to diabetes. Dietary fibre (sugar beet pulp, gum arabic, FOS) may be useful in the management of dogs and cats diagnosed with mild hyperglycemia (Nelson, 1989). In the small intestine, viscous NSPs act as a barrier to the release of nutrients and slow their absorption, which is important in the control of glucose and insulin metabolism. Blunted glycemia may occur by prolonging gastric emptying and intestinal transit time, slowing starch hydrolysis, and delaying glucose absorption.

Positive effects of fibre in petfood: Obesity and diabetes in cats and dogs, dental disease in dogs and hairball symptoms in cats and other negative health issues have been shown to be mitigated with fibrous diets. Fibre is associated with digestive (colonic) health and faecal regularity.

Innovative Fibre Sources

There is a growing consumer discontent with beet pulp and as absolute resistance to wheat bran, maize bran or soyhulls [Greg Aldrich (President of Pet Food & Ingredient Technology Inc., USA), 2013]. The potential alternative fibre ingredients are pea fibre, oat fibre, tomato pomace and fruit/ vegetable fibre (apple, carrot, pomegranate, etc.). Fibre from whole foods such as beans is excellent; beans have 22-24% total dietary fibre with about six % soluble fibre on DMB. Pea fibre (coat-and-hull dry process pea fibre and wet process cotyledon-based pea fibre) from the both the sources are high in insoluble fibre (more than 75%) with 5 to 25% as soluble fibre.

Tomato pomace is dried mixture of tomato skins, pulp and crushed seeds. It has 25-35% crude fibre, 281mg/kg lycopene, 224 ppm vitamin E and 2059 ppm total mixed tocopherols. Lycopene is the pigment responsible for tomato's red colour and it persists through processing. All these micronutrients are health promoting. Inclusion of tomato pomace at 1% of the diet, along with other antioxidant fruits and vegetables, aided cognitive function retention in older dogs (Milgram et al., 2005). It is commonly incorporated in dry formulas at 3-7% level.

Fat Content of Diets for Dogs

Dogs can be maintained by feeding dry-type diets containing 5 to 8 % total fat in dry matter (including 1% of the diet as linoleic acid), and many canned foods for adult maintenance contain in excess of 10 % on a DM basis. However, in practice, a minimal fat content of 5 % of DM has been suggested for commercial foods.

Although these concentrations appear sufficient for normal physiological functions, higher concentrations of fat may be desirable in practical dog foods to enhance acceptability and to improve hair coat sheen and help to prevent dermatitis. If such increases are made, the concentrations of other nutrients should be appropriately increased to maintain a satisfactory nutrient - to - energy ratio.

In extruded products, fat added above the 6% level can restrict the desired 'puffing' of starches and development of lamellar soy protein textures. In steam pelleted products, more than 4% added fat may provide too much lubrication in the die and reduce pellet cohesion.

Fat Content of Diets for Cats

Large cats in the wild may obtain 60 % of their energy from dietary fat, and diets containing 67 % ME as fat are efficiently utilized (Scott, 1968).

In domestic cats, reasonably high-fat diets from either animal or plant sources have been fed using purified diets containing 25-30 % total fat and 30-40 % protein. By comparison, dry-type, extruded cat foods typically contain 8 to 13 % fat DM. Both type and amount of dietary fat affect food acceptability to cats. Generally, higher-fat diets appear to be more palatable than low-fat diets. Beef tallow was selected over butter and chicken fat, but no preference was evident among beef tallow, lard, or partially hydrogenated vegetable oil (Kane et al., 1981). The recommended safe upper limit (SUL) of total dietary fat is approximately 70 % ME (82.5g per 1,000 kcal), although practical diets generally have 22 to 55 % ME, depending on cat food category.

Essentiality of arachidonic acid for cats: An important difference exists between the cat and the dog here. It has been reported that the cat has limited activity of certain desaturase enzymes involved in EFA metabolism, and a dietary requirement for a derived EFA, arachidonic acid has been established for cats. In reality this means cat has a requirement for animal fat and this is one of the factors contributing to the nature of the cat as an obligate carnivore.

Essential Fatty Acid Deficiency in Pets

Essential fatty acids maintain functional integrity of cell membranes, particularly in controlling the loss of water and are precursors of prostaglandins and leucotrienes. Lack of essential fatty acids may result in poor reproductive efficiency, poor wound healing, and a dry lustreless coat and scaly skin. If deficiency persists, lesions may develop in the external ear canal, between the toes, or in other 'hot spots' on the body.

Energy Deficiency and Excess in Dogs and Cats

The most conspicuous and reliable sign of simple energy deficiency is a generalized loss of body weight. Under conditions of partial or complete starvation, most internal organs exhibit some atrophy. A loss of subcutaneous, mesenteric, perirenal, uterine, testicular, and retroperitoneal fat is an early sign. Low fat content of the marrow in the long bones is a good indicator of prolonged energy deficiency. Brain size is least affected, but the size of gonads may be greatly decreased. Hypoplasia of lymph nodes, spleen, and thymus also observed. The adrenal glands are usually enlarged. The young skeleton is extremely sensitive to energy deficiency; growth may be slowed or stopped completely. In the adult, the skeleton may become osteoporotic. Lactation and the ability to perform work are also impaired. As muscle proteins are catabolized for energy, endogenous nitrogen losses increase. Parasitism and bacterial infections frequently occur under such circumstances and may superimpose other clinical signs. Signs of energy deficiency are frequently nonspecific, and diagnosis may be complicated by a simultaneous shortage of several nutrients.

Excess energy leads to overweight or even obesity. All body fat stores increase in size. Obesity may be linked to a number of diseases such as diabetes mellitus. It may enhance the severity of other diseases such as skeletal or heart problems as well as the risk of hyperlipidemia in cats. In growing animals, excess energy intake may induce excessive growth rates. In puppies from large breeds, this has been repeatedly associated with the onset or enhancement of developmental skeletal disease. It has been demonstrated in dogs that overfeeding from weaning to old age considerably impairs health and longevity (Kealy et al., 2002); hip dysplasia and osteoarthritis are common in overfed dogs. (See page No 34 for the role of fibre in weight management of dogs and cats).

Protein

Digestibility and Bioavailability of Protein and Amino Acids

Digestion of dietary protein by animals involves enzymatic cleavage of the protein to amino acids and small peptide residues that are capable of being absorbed by the mucosal cells of the small intestine. Protein digestibility – or more specifically, total digestive tract digestibility – is generally defined as the percentage of ingested protein that is not excreted in the faeces as measured by input and output of nitrogen. Bioavailability is generally defined as the degree to which an ingested nutrient in a particular source is absorbed in a form that can be utilized in the animal's metabolism (Lewis and Bayley, 1995). Much detailed work has been done on the bioavailability of amino acids from common proteins in food-animal nutrition using ileal digestibilities as a measure of bioavailability. Similar studies have been done with dogs; however, almost nothing is available for cats, perhaps because of the perceived difficulty in keeping ileally-cannulated cats (Mawby et al., 1999).

The first approach in determining bioavailability is to measure "apparent digestibility" of protein in a diet. This provides an overall evaluation of nitrogen absorbed but does not provide a measure of the "quality" or efficiency of utilization of nitrogen or of the individual essential amino acids. Historically, in human and animal nutrition, protein quality tests such as protein efficiency ratio (PER), biological value (BV), and net protein utilization (NPU), as determined in rat assays, have been used as one measure of overall amino acid bioavailability. Net protein utilization provides a measure of the efficiency of utilization of a protein.

Species differences: The apparent total tract digestibility of protein is similar in rats, cats, and dogs for highly digestible proteins. Proteins with lower digestibilities have higher apparent digestibilities in dogs than in cats.

Differences in efficiencies of utilization of the same protein in various species may result from different digestibilities and/or nitrogen and amino acid requirements. Carnivores in general, including cats, have lower apparent digestibilities of poorly digestible proteins and higher requirements for some amino acids such as arginine. Further refinement of the bioavailability values for individual amino acids results from determination of the ileal digestibility of the individual essential amino acids. Although these values provide a better indication of bioavailability than total gastrointestinal (GI) tract digestibility, dietary protein could be 100 percent digested and absorbed, but protein and amino acids would still enter the colon because of gastrointestinal secretions (sloughed mucosa and digestive enzymes). Thus, "true" ileal digestibilities have been measured using a number of techniques to estimate endogenous protein excreted from the ileum (Moughan et al., 1998). Since only some of this endogenous protein is essential for protein utilization, even true digestibilities of nitrogen and essential amino acids may not reflect true bioavailabilities. It should be noted that some dietary proteins contain inhibitors of trypsin or other enzymes that can greatly increase the loss of secreted enzymes.

Generally, some *in vivo* measure, such as weight gain and/or nitrogen retention, is considered the ultimate or "gold standard" for determining nitrogen and amino acid bioavailabilities (Lewis and Bayley, 1995).

Why do Cats Require Higher Protein?

It has been established that the cat has a higher requirement for protein than dog. Cat being an obligate carnivore use much of the protein in a normal meat diet to meet its energy requirements. Consequently, liver enzymes that deaminate amino acids in cats have a very high, constant activity rate and their activity is not modified even when the cat is receiving a low protein diet. But in omnivores and herbivores the activity of the enzymes is modulated and varies directly with the dietary protein content.

While most animals can survive on a minimal protein intake of 4 to 8% of the total dietary calories, the cat needs 18 to 20% of total calories as protein for growth as kittens and 12 to 13% for maintenance as adults. Adult cat needs 11 essential amino acids. Three others *viz.* cystein, glycine and serine probably are needed by the growing kitten for maximal growth.

The Need for Taurine in the Cats

Taurine is one of eleven essential amino acids required by cats. (Taurine is not an α-amino acid but β-amino sulphonic acid). While most mammals are able to synthesize taurine from sulfur containing amino acids, the cat's ability to synthesize taurine is very limited.

Furthermore, most other species are able to conjugate glycine with bile acids to form glycocholic acid. Cats, however, must use taurine for this conjugation process, forming taurocholic acid. The result is a large proportional loss of taurine in the bile. So cats require a constant dietary intake of taurine to maintain adequate tissue levels. Taurine is found in relatively high concentrations in a variety of tissues, including muscle, retina and the central nervous system (CNS). It is essentially absent from plant materials. The requirement for this nutrient is another example making the cat an obligate carnivore.

Deficiency Symptoms of Taurine

1. Reproductive function: Low plasma taurine concentrations can be responsible for fetal abortion and resorption, low birth rates and unthrifty kittens.
2. Degeneration of the retina: Feline central retinal degeneration (FCRD) is a progressive degeneration of the photoreceptor cells. The consequent blindness is irreversible.
3. Taurine deficiency causes dilated cardiomyopathy. This can be reversed by supplementing taurine at 500mg/day. The recommended levels are 1000 mg/kg DM for dry foods and 2000mg/kg DM for

canned products. It is known that fibre can bind taurine availability. As a result, cats on a high fibre diet as part of a weight control programme may require higher dietary taurine levels.

Amino Acid Imbalances and Antagonisms in Dogs and Cats

Omnivores and herbivores: Omnivores are most sensitive to disproportional quantities of dietary amino acids when fed diets limiting in protein and all of the essential amino acids (Harper et al., 1970). Omnivores and herbivores adapt to high-protein diets by decreasing their food intake and weight gain for 1-5 days (depending on the levels of dietary protein used). Amino acid and nitrogen homeostasis is restored thereafter, by up-regulating amino acid and nitrogen catabolic enzymes; normal growth resumes. It is clear that cats are much less sensitive to disproportional quantities of dietary amino acids than are rats, chicks, and other herbivores and omnivores (Rogers et al., 1987).

Carnivores: Although the metabolic basis of the high crude protein requirement for maintenance (for cats) is controversial (Rogers and Morris, 2002; Russell et al., 2002), it has been shown consistently that cats will not maintain nitrogen balance at the same low dietary crude protein concentrations that occur for most herbivores and omnivores (Hendriks et al., 1997). It is known that cats do not up- or down-regulate the nitrogen catabolic enzymes to nearly the same extent as omnivores and herbivores, so it appears that cats are always adapted to handle a medium to high level of dietary amino acids (Table-3). This minimizes the adverse effects of disproportional quantities of amino acids.

Table-3. Crude protein and essential amino acid requirements (Recommended Allowance; g per 1000 kcal ME) of the growing puppies and kittens*

Amino acid	Growing puppies (4–14 weeks old)	Growing puppies (14 weeks & older)	Growing kittens
Crude protein, g	56.3	43.8	56.3
Arginine (g)	1.98	1.65	2.4
Histidine (g)	0.98	0.63	0.83
Isoleucine (g)	1.63	1.25	1.4
Methionine (g)	0.88	0.65	1.1
Methionine & Cystine (g)	1.75	1.33	2.2
Leucine (g)	3.22	2.05	3.2

Lysine (g)	2.20	1.75	2.1
Phenylalanine (g)	1.63	1.25	1.3
Phenylalanine & Tyrosine (g)	3.25	2.50	4.8
Threonine (g)	2.03	1.58	1.6
Tryptophan (g)	0.58	0.45	0.40
Valine (g)	1.70	1.40	1.6
Taurine (g)	–	–	0.10

* Adapted from Nutrient requirements of dogs and cats (NRC, 2006)

Only a very minor growth depression occurred in kittens when crude protein was increased in a diet limiting in threonine (Hammer et al., 1996a), whereas Strieker (1991) showed that, even if methionine was limiting, increasing dietary crude protein slightly increased weight gain. When methionine was severely limiting, it caused severe pyrodermatitis at the commisures of the mouth and necrolytic dermatosis on the pads of the feet, all of which were rapidly corrected when more methionine was added to the diet.

Cats are also insensitive to arginine-lysine antagonisms and much less sensitive to leucine-isoleucine and-valine antagonism. Thus, cats transitorily reduced their food intake and growth when excess leucine was added to the diet only if isoleucine was already limiting, and even then, cats would select the high-leucine diet over the more balanced diets.

Lysine-arginine Antagonism in Dogs

Although 10 or 20 g of extra free lysine per kg diet had no effect, 40 g excess lysine in the diet caused a growth depression and classical clinical signs of arginine deficiency (emesis, increased plasma ammonia, and orotic aciduria) when the diet contained 4 g arginine/kg. An additional 4g arginine prevented the clinical signs and improved weight gain but did not appear to fully restore it. The excess lysine caused a generalized amino aciduria. The SUL for lysine is >20 and <40 g per kg diet containing 4.0 kcal ME per g.

Metabolic adaptation of amino acid metabolism in dogs indicates that they are intermediate between rats and cats. Results of the studies during the past 50 years indicated that dogs show amino acid imbalances and antagonisms more similar to those of rats. In general, dogs appear to be more sensitive to disproportionalities among dietary amino acids than cats, especially when fed low-protein diets.

Diets based on high levels of starch are often limited by the amount of lysine and has to be supplemented. At the other extreme, excessive lysine relative to arginine can create an antagonism interfering with normal urea cycle function resulting in amino aciduria, a potentially lethal condition.

Interestingly, this antagonism has been exploited as a therapy for feline herpes virus (FHV-1) sufferers by providing high dose oral L-lysine to intentionally antagonize the high arginine appetite for the disease.

Minerals

Dogs and cats essentially require six major minerals (Ca, P, Mg, Na, K and Cl) and six micro minerals (Fe, Cu, Zn, Mn, I and Se). Minerals serve many physiological functions as protective, structural, regulatory and general metabolic functions (Readers may refer Principles of animal nutrition and feed technology Textbook for details).

Calcium to Phosphorus Levels

The adult dogs and cats need 0.5% and 0.59% calcium and 0.4% and 0.5% phosphorus while growing and reproducing dogs and cats require 1.0% and 1.0% calcium and 0.9% and 0.84% phosphorus. Sources of fresh meat, poultry and fish can supply a Ca: P of 1:15 - 20. Feeding of such incorrectly balanced diets based on fresh meat result in calcium deficiency. Young, fast-growing animals are affected. Eclampsia, nutritional secondary hyperparathyroidism (NSH) are noticed as a consequence.

The bioavailability of trace-elements is reduced by a high content of certain minerals (e.g., calcium), the level of other trace elements (e.g., high zinc level decreases copper absorption) and sources of phytic acid (plant feedstuffs). Hence as the calcium level approaches the stated nutritional maximum, it may be necessary to increase the levels of certain trace elements such as zinc and copper.

High intake of calcium has an adverse effect on skeletal development in large breed dogs, particularly during the early growth phase. Therefore a strict nutritional maximum is recommended for foods intended for large breed puppies. Feeding high calcium diets is often held responsible for contributing to bone problems in young, rapidly growing (large breed) dogs.

Potassium

Potassium deficiency in the body is most often due to an excessive loss rather than too little dietary intake (Potassium is widely distributed in many plant foods). Like sodium and chloride, potassium deficiency can occur in animals that that have chronic diarrhoea and/ or vomiting, burns, kidney disease, etc illnesses, which result in a loss of potassium from the body.

Potassium toxicity generally does not occur from excessive intake as long as the kidneys are functioning normally. The potassium level in the blood, however, can reach a dangerous level in a disease called hypoadrenocorticism or Addison's disease. This is a disease in which the adrenal gland does not produce enough of the hormone that helps regulate the amounts of potassium in the blood.

Iron

Dog diets need iron at 80 mg per each kg. A deficiency in iron results in the development of anaemia leading to decreased growth rate, weakness, and increased susceptibility to stress or disease. Animal with iron deficiency may also develop constipation.

Zinc

Zinc is one of the essential minerals that need supplementation in diets for dogs and cats. Deficiency may be due to a lack of sufficient zinc in the diet or to a decreased bioavailability. There are several factors that affect the absorption of zinc. Some breeds have an inability to adequately absorb zinc and they must be fed a diet that is higher in zinc to prevent zinc deficiency-associated skin problems. Fibre and phytates bind zinc and reduce its absorption. Therefore, animals that are fed a diet high in plant feedstuffs may have an increased risk of developing zinc deficiencies. Similarly, high calcium level in the diet binds the zinc causing zinc deficiency. Dogs or cats with inflammatory bowel disease may develop zinc deficiency because of lack of absorption. Zinc deficiency in the dog most commonly occurs as a skin condition is called 'zinc responsive dermatosis'

Requirements of Cats for Water

As fundamentally desert animals, cats have developed adaptations to accommodate periods of water unavailability. Their greater ability to concentrate urine than dogs, humans, and many other species allows them to mitigate insensible losses. Cats also appear to be able to tolerate dehydration better than most species (NRC, 1986). As a result, the requirement for water may be lower for cats than for dogs.

4

Diet Formulation for Dogs and Cats

Process of Diet Formulation

The actual process of diet formulation involves the following:

1. Note down the requirements for the animal
2. Select the ingredients in specific amounts that furnish the required and available nutrients to the diets

Diet formulation may be done by either hand formulation or computer formulation. Now-a-days all commercial companies and consulting nutritionists use a computer-based process known as "linear programming." The value of linear programming is that it can deal with the vast array of ingredients, nutrient requirements, and restrictions in just a few seconds.

Dogs and cats have a demonstrated requirement for specific nutrients but not a requirement for specific feedstuffs to be included in their diet (AAFCO, 2002). Nevertheless, pets can be quite individualistic in their feeding habits and often exhibit food preferences favouring a particular form (forms of food: dry, semimoist, canned) or texture (mixed; soft-moist; dry; flavour induced by specific ingredients, e.g., fish).

Dogs: Dogs differ from cats in that they are not strict carnivores but fall more in the omnivorous category. This fact allows a great deal more latitude in ingredient selection and formulation. It is entirely feasible to formulate an adequate dog diet using no animal tissue-based ingredients. This fact and the remarkable adaptability of the dog have led to the successful use of commercial diets that differ widely in their ingredient composition, texture, and form.

Cats: While cats are true carnivores in the wild, most commercial diets for domestic cats contain significant amounts of vegetable matter that is

45

satisfactorily used by the animal as a nutrient source. However, animal tissue-based ingredients contribute significantly to the acceptability of the food by the cat and, therefore, play a role in adequate consumption. Animal source feedstuffs (meat byproducts, fish, eggs, milk) should be included up to 30-40 %. When feeding meat, it is important that all of the bone has been chopped to prevent pieces of bone from becoming lodged in the throat or digestive system; either raw or cooked meat can be fed. Sometimes there may be digestive trouble. Provide vegetables, green grass to avoid digestive trouble. Green grass helps to expel fur balls from the stomach.

Acceptable commercial cat diets contain a portion of animal source ingredients to meet specific nutrient requirements (e.g., arachidonic acid, taurine, vitamin A) if not met by synthetic sources. Generally speaking, strict vegetarian diets, when fed alone, are not nutritionally adequate for cats, even though such diets can be made sufficiently palatable to be readily consumed.

Nutrient Requirements of Dogs

The nutrient requirements (NRC, 2006) are given here in nutshell for easy application.

ME Requirements per day per kg $W^{0.75}$

Maintenance	130 Kcal
Growing	260 Kcal
Adolescence	200 Kcal
Pregnancy	186 Kcal
Lactation	460 Kcal

Fat requirement per day per kg $W^{0.75}$

Maintenance	1.8 g
Growth	up to 5.9 g

Protein requirement per day per kg $W^{0.75}$

Maintenance	3.28 g
Growth	up to 15.7 g

Feeding of Dogs

FEDIAF (2011) specified the minimum recommended nutrient levels for dog foods. A standard balanced adult dog food should contain 18% crude protein, 5.5% fat, 3.5-6% crude fibre, 1.32% linoleic acid, 0.5% Ca and 0.4% P on dry matter basis. It should also be balanced with essential nutrients, minerals and vitamins.

A standard balanced dog food for early growth and reproduction should contain 25% crude protein, 8.5% fat, 3.5-6% crude fibre, 1.30% linoleic acid, 0.03% arachidonic acid, 0.08% alpha-linolenic acid, 0.05% EPA+DHA, 1.0% Ca and 0.9% P on dry matter basis. It should also be balanced with essential nutrients, minerals and vitamins.

Feeding During Pregnancy

Irrespective of the breed of the dog, the female should be at least one year of age and it should be in 'the second heat-period' before she is bred. The nutrient requirements of the female during the first 6 to 7 weeks of pregnancy are not higher than for dogs at maintenance. It is recommended to feed extra energy to start four weeks after mating. The bitch's feed intake should be increased gradually so that at the time of whelping her daily intake is approximately 25% to 50% higher than her normal maintenance needs, depending on the size of the litter and size of the bitch. Her body weight should increase by approximately 15% to 25% by the time of whelping (from 15 kg to 17-19 kg).

During the last 2 to 3 weeks, requirements for all nutrients will increase. Normally pregnant dog will eat more during this phase. The diet has to be offered several times each day. Mammary gland development and milk production occur 1 to 5 days before parturition. As whelping nears, the female may lose her appetite. This is considered normal behaviour. In many cases, food refusal during the 9th week is an indication that whelping will occur within the next 24 to 48 hours. Usually within 24 hours after whelping the female's appetite will return. Fresh water in a clean bowl should be available at all times. Keeping water bowls clean and changing water frequently tend to encourage water consumption.

Feeding During Lactation

Milk production is one of the most nutritionally demanding stages in a female's life. The demand for milk by nursing puppies will continue to increase for about 20 to 30 days. Consequently, the female's food and water requirements increase during this time. At peak lactation, the female's food intake may be two to four times above her maintenance food intake. Puppies will start nibbling solid food at 2 and half a week age.

Acclimatizing puppies to a good quality diet at an early stage will help prevent finicky eaters. Normally puppies are weaned between 6 and 8 weeks of age. By this time, the female's food consumption should be less than 50% above her maintenance level. To help reduce the milk flow and prevent mummery gland problems, the following procedure for weaning is recommended.

On the day of weaning, the mother should not receive any food, but should have plenty of fresh water to drink. On the second day, the dam should receive 1/4 the amount of food she was fed prior to being bred. The dam and puppies can be grouped together for several hours so that the pups can nurse the dam dry. On the third day, the dam should receive 1/2 the amount fed prior to breeding, and on the fourth day, 3/4 the amount. By the fifth day she should be offered her usual maintenance level of food. If the litter is large, the female may be quite thin when the puppies are weaned. In this case, she should be given extra food after the fifth day weaning until her body condition returns to normal.

Newborn Puppies and Kittens

The neonatal period is considered to be the first two weeks after birth. The offspring of dogs and cats are altricial. That is they are born in a relatively immature state and are completely dependent upon their mother's care. The first 36 hours of their life are very critical. A quiet, warm whelping area should be provided.

Colostrum Feeding

The dog and cat have an endotheliochorial placenta consisting of four layers. This type of placenta allows only about 10 to 20% of passive immunity to be transferred *in utero*. Therefore, puppies and kittens have to acquire the major proportion of passive immunity after birth through the colostrum. The time during which the newborn's gastrointestinal tract (GIT) is permeable to the intact immunoglobulins in colostrum is very short (about the first 48 hours of life).

Feeding of Puppies

Under normal conditions newborn puppies are nursed by their mother through natural teat feeding and they learn to eat mother's food after opening eyes at about 7 to 10 days of age. The ME content of bitch milk is 126 kcal while that of queen is 97 kcal / 100 g (Table 1). In healthy puppies and kittens, the dam's milk (900-1700 g in German Shepherds to 100-180 g in Dachshund) supports normal growth until the young are 3 to 4 weeks old. The GIT of newborn puppies are uniquely suited to digest and absorb the milk produced by the mother. The ingestion of milk is a potent stimulator for enteric growth and for the development of the intestinal mucosal cells.

Table 1. Composition of milks of farm animals, bitch and queen (g/100ml)

	Cow	Goat	Ewe	Sow	Bitch	Queen
Protein	3.4	3.4	5.5	5.8	7.5	9.1
Fat	3.7	4.5	7.4	8.5	8.3	3.7
Lactose	4.8	4.1	4.8	4.8	3.7	4.9
Calcium	0.12	0.13	0.16	0.25	0.29	0.04
Phosphorus	0.09	0.11	0.13	0.17	0.24	0.07
Magnesium	0.012	0.02	0.017	0.02	–	–
Total solids (Fat + S.N.F)	12.7	13.2	19.3	20.5	22.6	17.8
ME, kcal/100g	61	65	–	–	126	97
Lactose,mg/kcal ME	77	62	28	71		

Note: On a caloric basis, the lactose content of cow's milk is nearly 3 times that of bitch's milk.

During this time, puppies double their birth weight and become increasingly more active. Sometimes special attention may be required to help them in case of some nervous or inattentive dams. Lactation period may last for more than 8 weeks but most of the dog breeders practice weaning at about 4, 6 or 8 weeks of age. Weaned puppies are gradually shifted to artificial feeding of milk-based semi-solid or liquid diets.

Nutritional Care of Orphan Puppies

An orphan is any young animal that does not have access to the milk or care of its mother. Orphaned animals (due to the death of the mother) must be kept in a warm and clean environment. Maintaining the appropriate temperature is of the utmost importance for the survivability of newborns. Sometimes mother is unable to nurse the puppies due to agalactia or mastitis. Such orphan puppies need artificial feeding from the very first day of life. Such puppies are usually deprived of mother's colostrum and they are more susceptible to infection requiring more hygienic care during feeding and watering.

Compare the composition of the milk of cow or buffalo that is available with that of the bitch. Puppies that are fed on cow milk will develop severe diarrhoea, because of higher level of lactose in cow's milk. It is better to prepare milk-replacer by combining milks and eggs. Eggs are added to increase the protein and dilute the lactose concentration of the milk.

For a litter of eight pups, about 600 ml of milk/day is sufficient for the first 3 days, after which they should receive 1.2 L. A milk (bitch milk) substitute may be prepared by adding 200 g cream to 800 ml cow milk along with one egg yolk, 6 g steamed bone meal, 2000 IU vitamin A, 500 IU vitamin D and 4 g citric acid.

Method of feeding: Bottle feeding is almost necessary in the first 2 weeks when eyes are not open. It can be done with the help of a large teat dropper or from a shallow pan. Puppies are to be trained to drink milk from shallow pans. The pup's muzzle should be pushed into the milk (lukewarm) until it learns to lap it up. It takes about 3-7 days to train the puppy to feed from a dish. A liquid feed containing about 25-30 per cent dry matter should be fed @ 14-16 per cent of body weight divided by the number of daily meals at each feeding, 12 times in the I week, 8 times in II week, 6 times in III & IV week followed by thrice daily feedings in day time only from the fifth week of age. At 5 or 6 weeks of age, the puppies should be weaned and receive cow's milk and solid food. It is well to wean them on the type of diet that they are to receive later.

Good quality starter diets are introduced to puppies at 3 - 4 weeks age. They can be easily prepared from milk and other foods at home. It should contain about 30-35 per cent protein and 30-35 per cent of edible fat and carbohydrates (starch, lactose and sugar). Adequate amount of minerals and vitamins are be added. Adequate nutrition is best demonstrated by maximal growth and production.

Feeding of Weaned Puppies

A liquid diet (about 30% DM) may be prepared by using cream, cereal flour, egg yolk and milk or milk powder. This is to be fed at the rate of 15% of BW at different intervals during the day. Young pups should be fed at least three times a day. Fresh water in a clean bowl should be available at all times. Establishing routine eating habits by feeding a puppy in the same place and at the same time each day is recommended. The amount of food offered to a pup will vary depending upon its size, activity, metabolism and environment. The daily requirement may be calculated at 50-55 g DM per kg body weight during the active growth up to about 6 months of age. Afterwards the quantity may be reduced to 38-40 g. Puppies should not be allowed to become overweight.

Proper feeding of young dogs supports normal muscle and skeletal development and a rate of growth that is typical for the dog's particular breed. The most rapid period of growth for all dogs occurs between 3 and 5 months of age. Overfeeding for maximal growth rate and early maturity should be avoided. Portion-controlled feeding is the recommended feeding regimen for growing dogs. A puppy's daily portion of food should be divided into three meals per day until the puppy is 4 to 6 months of age, after 6 months, two meals per day can be fed and once a day when they are eight months or older.

Dry foods are often preferred compared to semimoist and canned foods for feeding adult animals for the following two reasons. Dry foods are less dense calorically, and they can also help to maintain proper tooth and gum hygiene. Dry foods are more economical and easier to feed.

Feeding schedule: From weaning to 12 weeks of age 4-5 times a day, 3-6 months thrice daily and 6 month onwards twice daily.

Feeding the Mature dog: The "maintenance" period is referred to the time after a dog has reached its full maturity. Mature dogs have the lowest (22 g DM) requirement. Feeding recommendations for adult dogs can vary depending upon the breed, activity. Whether or not an animal is fed once or twice each day, it should be fed at the same time. Fresh drinking water should always be made available.

Feeding Hardworking Dogs

Hardworking dogs are usually referred to as those used for hunting, herding sheep, or sled dog racing, as well as dogs who routinely run long distances (i.e., greater than 32 km per week). The more active a dog, the more food it requires. This applies regardless of the seasonal environmental temperature or a dog's physiological state. All nutrients will be required in greater amounts than for an adult dog at maintenance. Physical activity is the outwardly visible result of a complex sequence of muscular contractions. The combustions of dietary fuels such as fat, protein and carbohydrate provide the energy for muscular work. Water, minerals and vitamins are involved in utilizing energy for work.

Working dogs may have increased nutrient needs when they are training or actually working. The requirement for additional nutrients will depend on an individual dog's activity level. During leisure days, it is recommended that the amount of the dog's training / working ration be reduced, or that the dog be gradually changed to a lower energy, less nutrient dense dog food. Maintaining dogs in good body condition in the off season will help make conditioning for training- / working-seasons less stressful.

Working dogs should not be fed a meal immediately before or immediately after a session of hard activity. Such may result in poor performance and gastric upset or discomfort as evidenced by vomiting or loose stools. Snacks or treats may be provided during periods of increased activity after a period of rest with fresh cool water and followed a period of rest. These snacks prevent hunger discomfort and fatigue in hard working dogs.

Balanced Diet Chart for Dogs

1. Growing puppy

Problem 1. Calculate the nutrient requirement of 5 kg growing (four months of age) German Shephard (Alsatian) dog and formulate a balanced diet.

Solution: Metabolic body weight: $5^{0.75}$ = 3.54 kg

Energy requirement (up to 50% of adult weight) = 210 kcal ME/kgW$^{0.75}$
(from Table No.1b Chapter 2)
Protein requirement (14 weeks and older puppies) = 12.2 g/ kgW$^{0.75}$
(from Table No.4 Chapter 2)
Requirements per day: Energy: 3.54 × 210 = 702 kcal ME
Protein: 3.54 × 12.20 = 40.8 g CP

Composition of ingredients, per 100 g			Balanced Diet I			Balanced Diet II		
Energy, kcal	Protein, g	Ingredient, g	Quantity, g	Ener, kcal	Prot, g	Quantity, g	Ener, kcal	Pro, g
67	3.2	Milk	300	201.0	9.60	200	134.00	6.40
143	11.3	Egg	100	143.0	11.30	50	71.50	5.65
346	11.8	Wheat	50	173.0	5.90	–	–	–
350	22.5	Pulses	50	175.0	11.25	–	–	–
49	4.7	Beans	50	24.50	2.35	–	–	–
194	19	Meat	–	–	–	125	242.50	23.75
345	6.8	Rice	–	–	–	75	258.75	5.10
				716.5	**40.4**		**706.75**	**40.90**

Note: Minerals and vitamins supplement need to be provided daily to meet their requirements.

Problem 2. Calculate the nutrient requirement of 2 kg growing (four months of age) Spitz dog and formulate a balanced diet.

Metabolic body weight: $2^{0.75}$ = 1.68 kg

Energy requirement (up to 50% of adult weight) = 210 kcal ME/kgW$^{0.75}$

Protein requirement (14 weeks and older puppies) = 12.2 g/ kgW$^{0.75}$

Requirements per day: Energy: 1.68 × 210= 353 kcal ME

Protein: 1.68 × 12.20= 20.52 g CP

Composition of ingredients, per 100 g			Balanced Diet I			Balanced Diet II		
Energy, kcal	Protein, g	Ingredient,	Quantity, g	Ener, kcal	Prot, g	Quantity, g	Ener, kcal	Prot, g
67	3.2	Milk	120	80.4	3.84	200	134.00	6.40
143	11.3	Egg	50	71.5	5.65	25	35.75	2.83
346	11.8	Wheat	40	138.4	4.72	–	–	–
350	22.5	Pulses	20	70.0	4.50	–	–	–
49	4.7	Beans	40	19.6	1.88	–	–	–
194	19	Meat	–	–	–	50	97.00	9.50
345	6.8	Rice	–	–	–	25	86.25	1.70
				379.9	**20.59**		**353.00**	**20.43**

Note: Minerals and vitamins supplement need to be provided daily to meet their requirements.

2. Adult dogs

Problem 3. Calculate the nutrient requirement of 25 kg adult (four years of age) German Shephard (Alsatian) dog and formulate a balanced diet.

Metabolic body weight: $25^{0.75} = 11.18$ kg

Energy requirement (3-7 years of age) = 115 kcal ME/kgW$^{0.75}$

(from Table No.3b Chapter 2)

Protein requirement (adults) = 3.28 g/ kgW$^{0.75}$

(from Table No.4 Chapter 2)

Requirements per day: Energy: $11.18 \times 115 = 1286$ kcal ME

Protein: $11.18 \times 3.28 = 37.0$ g CP

Composition of ingredients, per 100 g			Balanced Diet I			Balanced Diet II		
Energy, kcal	Protein, g	Ingredient,	Quantity, g	Ener, kcal	Protein, g	Quantity, g	Ener, kcal	Protein, g
67	3.2	Milk	275	184.25	8.80	150	100.50	4.80
345	6.8	Rice	280	966.00	19.04	250	862.50	17.00
350	22.5	Pulses	25	87.50	5.63	–	–	–
48	0.9	Carrot	50	24.00	0.45	–	–	–
49	4.7	Beans	60	29.40	2.82	–	–	–
346	11.8	Wheat	–	–	–	70	242.20	8.26
194	19.0	Meat	–	–	–	40	77.60	7.60
				1291.5	**36.74**		**1282.8**	**37.66**

Note: Minerals and vitamins supplement need to be provided daily to meet their requirements.

Problem 4. Calculate the nutrient requirement of 8 kg adult (four years of age) Spitz dog and formulate a balanced diet.

Metabolic body weight = 4.76 kg

Energy requirement (3-7 years of age) = 115 kcal ME ME/kgW$^{0.75}$

Protein requirement (adults) = 3.28 g/ kgW$^{0.75}$

Requirements per day: Energy: 4.76 × 115= 547 kcal ME

Protein: 4.76 × 3.28 = 15.6 g CP

Composition of ingredients, per 100 g			Balanced Diet I			Balanced Diet II		
Energy, kcal	Protein, g	Ingredient,	Quantity, g	Energy, kcal	Protein, g	Quantity, g	Energy, kcal	Protein, g
67	3.2	Milk	100	67.00	3.20	100	67.00	3.20
350	22.5	Pulses	20	70.00	4.50	–	–	–
48	0.9	Carrot	20	9.60	0.18	–	–	–
194	19	Meat	–	–	–	25	48.50	4.75
345	6.8	Rice	120	414.00	8.16	125	431.25	8.50
				560.60	**16.04**		**546.75**	**16.45**

Note: Minerals and vitamins supplement need to be provided daily to meet their requirements.

A balanced ration for Border Security Force dogs

Ingredient	Quantity per day*
Rice /Wheat grain	480 g
Dog biscuit	30 g
Vegetables, fresh	230 g
Meat dressed with bones	680 g

* Dogs are supplemented with calcium gluconate tablet, multivitamin tablet and shark liver oil as per the need.

Feeding Schedule for dogs: A guide chart

Body weight kg	Cereals g	Meat* g	Milk g
2–5	100-200	50-100	125-150
5–10	200-300	100-200	150-250
10–20	300-500	200-400	250-400

* The 'meat' portion of the diet may be completely avoided by including 1-2 eggs and pulses / oilseed meals. Vegetables may also be added to meet the requirement of fibre and micronutrients.

Vegetarian Diets for Dogs

Though dogs are meat liking animals they can survive on a vegetarian diet. Vegetarian diets should be formulated with care to ensure that all the nutrients are provided to meet the requirements. If we consider the advantages of a vegetarian diet for dogs, it is only advantageous to the owner of the pet, if he/she is a vegetarian. That is without hurting the sentiments, the pet owner can proudly raise his/her pet dog on a vegetarian diet. Nutritionally balanced diets can be formulated without meat and eggs. But how for your pet, a meat liking animal is pleased!

The way to a man's heart is through his stomach. So dog is no different from man in this aspect. Feed your dog well and get closer to its heart.

Dog is a very intelligent animal with emotional thinking. It has a smelling power as well as learning capability 40 times more than the human being. Whenever some non-vegetarian stuff is cooked in the neighbourhood, your pet will be facing temptation, mental agony and torture. That is why the vegetarian diet given to dogs should contain eggs.

Feeding Management

Dogs may be fed successfully in a number of ways. These include portion-control feeding, free-choice or *ad libitum* feeding and timed feeding (Pattanaik, 2012). Portion-control feeding is followed in adult animals, obese animals and in animals that might overeat if fed free-choice. Most nursing mothers and growing animals are fed by free-choice feeding. Timed feeding method involves making a portion of feed available for the pet to eat for a specified period of time (for example, 30 minutes) and removing the bowl after the scheduled-time, even if the food is not consumed.

Feeding of Cats

Of all the animals domesticated by man, cat has the most unusual and most complicated nutritional requirements. Feline metabolism has evolved into that of an obligate carnivore i.e the cat has adapted its metabolism to efficient utilization of a strictly carnivorous diet.

Peculiar Aspects of Feline Nutrition

1. Cat has a shorter small intestine, lack of caecum with bacterial flora and generally shorter transit time. Feline intestine is adapted for a high-fat, high-protein diet, that is, high-energy, low-bulk diet.

2. Cat is somewhat peculiar in its attitude toward food and its eating behaviour. Cats tend to eat and drink limited quanities on numerous occasions when fed *ad libitum*.
3. Cats are unable to synthesize arachidonic acid from linoleic acid. So arachidonic acid must be supplied by animal fat in the diet.
4. Taurine must be supplied in the form of dietary meat, poultry or fish products, because of the limited ability of the feline liver to synthesize taurine.
5. Protein requirement of the cat is the highest. Cats need two to three times more protein than most other animals under comparable circumstances. Cat is unique in its failure to curtail protein-catabolising enzymes when fed a low-protein diet.
6. Cat has higher dietary requirements for arginine and niacin. Cat is unable to synthesize arginine. In the absence of dietary arginine, the usual high catabolism of protein generates a load of ammonia that cannot be detoxified by its incorporation into urea and hyperammonemia develops.

   The process of obtaining niacin from tryptophan is not available in the cat though it possesses all the necessary enzymes. This is due to a high level of activity of the enzyme picolinic carboxylase, which effectively diverts tryptophan conversion via the alternate pathway away from niacin.
7. Cats lack the enzyme necessary to cleave β-carotene. It is dependent on a dietary source of preformed vitamin A.

Formulation of Balanced Diets for Cats

FEDIAF (2011) specified the minimum recommended nutrient levels for cat foods. A standard balanced adult cat food should contain 25% crude protein, 9.0% fat, 3.5-6% crude fibre, 0.5% linoleic acid, 0.006% arachidonic acid, 0.59% Ca and 0.5% P on dry matter basis. It should also be balanced with essential nutrients, minerals and vitamins.

A standard balanced cat food for growth and reproduction should contain 28-30 % crude protein, 9.0 % fat, 3.5-6 % crude fibre, 0.55 % linoleic acid, 0.02 % arachidonic acid, 0.02 % alpha-linolenic acid, 0.01% EPA+DHA, 1.0% Ca and 0.84% P on dry matter basis. It should also be balanced with essential nutrients, minerals and vitamins.

In general, most cats given the adequate opportunity for exercise under a variety of environmental options (e.g., roaming outdoors) they learn to regulate their food intake and maintain a relative lean body mass. Cats can adapt to a single daily meal after reaching adult stage. In case of overweight cats, feed restriction has to be followed.

Pregnant or lactating cats and kittens require an *ad libitum* feeding arrangement to allow for adequate food intake during the energy- dependant physiologic processes of pregnancy, lactation and growth.

Feeding During Pregnancy

The weight gain pattern that occurs in pregnant queens is slightly different from that observed in bitches. Pregnant queens exhibit a linear increase in weight beginning around the second week of gestation in contrast to bitches where the weight increase occurs during the last third of gestation. In dogs, almost all of the pre-parturition gain is lost at whelping. In contrast, weight loss immediately following parturition in the cat accounts for only 40% of the weight that was gained during pregnancy. The remaining 60% of the queen's weight gain is body fat and is gradually lost during lactation. Thus it appears that the queen is able to prepare for the excessive demands of lactation by accumulating surplus body energy stores during gestation.

Litter size is positively influenced by the provision of adequate fat in the queen's diet, and fat in the diet should provide optimal levels of EFAs, particularly arachidonic acid. Taurine is also an important nutrient to consider because both conception rate and kitten birth weight are reduced in queens when dietary taurine is limiting.

The diet must supply essential nutrients in the proper balance for the developing kittens and prepare the female for the stress of lactation. Throughout gestation, the female may show a slow, steady increase in body weight and at the same time a gradual increase in food intake beginning the second week of gestation and continuing until parturition. Hormonal and behavioural changes that occur during reproduction may cause periods of undereating, overeating or noteating. For example, many queens undergo a short period of partial appetite loss at about the 3rd week of gestation, lasting anywhere from 3 to 10 days. During the last trimester of pregnancy, requirement for nutrients will increase. Diet has to be offered several times. As littering nears, a female may also lose her appetite. Feed refusal during the 9th week of gestation is frequently a good indication that littering will occur within the next 1 or 2 days. Usually within 24 hrs after delivery the female's appetite will slowly increase.

At the end of gestation, the queen should be receiving approximately 25% to 50% more food than her normal maintenance needs. The queen's weight gain should be monitored closely to prevent excessive weight gain during this time. Queens typically gain between 12% and 38% of their pre-pregnancy body weight by the end of gestation.

Feeding During Lactation

The demand for milk by nursing kittens will continue to about 20 to 30 days. Consequently, the female's food and water requirements increase during this time. They have to be fed two or three times per day. Fresh water should be made available. Newborn kittens typically quadruple their body weight in the first month of life, which reemphasizes the extreme nutritional demands placed on the nursing queen.

Kittens start nibbling solid food. When kittens are 3 to 4 weeks of age, interest in solid food begins and the dam's interest in nursing declines. Weaning of kittens usually takes place between 6 and 8 weeks of age.

For females that continue to maintain significant milk production, mammary congestion and discomfort can be a problem. Resolution of this problem may be hastened by limit-feeding the queen according to the similar procedure as mentioned in case of bitch.

Feeding of Kittens

Help the kittens to suckle the dam. In an emergency, like mother's inability to nurse their kittens due to agalactia or mastitis and for orphan kittens artificial feeding is required from the very first day of life. Kittens have to be trained to drink cow/buffalo milk-based feed consisting of egg yolk, cereal flour, cream, minerals and vitamins. Orphans are to be fed at the rate of 10-15% of BW/day at birth. This gradually increases to 20-25%. They should be fed four times daily by 2 months age. After each feeding, the stomach of kitten should be rubbed with coarse warm towel. Kittens start nibbling the solid food of the dam from 3rd or 4th week of age.

Feeding of Weaned Kittens

Kittens should be weaned by 6 to 8 weeks of age. Kittens require higher levels of protein than pups. It is recommended that kittens be fed two to three times a day during this period of rapid growth (up to 6 months of age). Kittens tend to be "occasional" eaters as they take a large number of small meals throughout the day. Too much noice, new surroundings, the cleanliness of food/water, dishes may all be the factors to consider if a kitten refuses to eat.

At 26 weeks of age, the growth rate starts to level off. The frequency of feeding may be two meals per day thereafter. However, kittens continue to develop inside with normal growth ending at about 12 months of age.

Feeding the Mature Cat

A cat can be fed a maintenance diet after it is one year of age. An adult cat with normal activity requires only a maintenance diet. Cats should be fed as individuals. Kittens from the same litter may acquire different tastes and eating habits. Because cats tend to be nibblers or "occasional eaters", they should have access to their food for several hours each day. Fresh clean water has to be made available. The cat has a reputation to be called as finicky eater. The estimated daily food (DM) intakes are given in Table 2.

Table 2. Estimated Daily Food Allowances for Cats

Cat	Weight of Cat (kg)	Food intake (90% DM; ME 3.2 kcal/g)	
		g/kg BW	g/Cat
Kitten			
10 Weeks	0.9-1.1	78	70-86
20 Weeks	1.9-2.5	41	78-103
30 Weeks	2.5-3.8	31	78-118
40 Weeks	2.9-3.8	25	73-95
Adult (50 Weeks of age or older) **			
Inactive	2.2-4.5	22	48-90
Active	2.2-4.5	25	55-113
Gestation	2.5-4.0	31	78-124
Lactaion*	2.2-4.0	78	172-312

* Queens nursing 4-5 kittens in week 6 of lactation;
** During pregnancy 1.25 to 1.5 times of maintenance ration can be given till the end of gestation; during lactation, it should be increased to 2 to 3.5 times of adult maintenance ration.

Balanced Diet Chart for Cat

Growing kitten

Problem 1. Calculate the nutrient requirement of 1 kg growing active cat (six months of age) and formulate a balanced diet.

Metabolic body weight: $1^{0.67} = 1$ kg
Energy requirement: Maintenance Energy Requirement (MER)
for active cat = 100 kcal ME/kg$W^{0.67}$; (from Table 10 Chapter 2)

ME requirement for cat of 4-9 months = 1.75 to 2.0 times of MER;

(from Table No.8b Chapter 2)

Protein requirement (growing kittens) = 11.80 g/ kgW$^{0.67}$

(from Table No.9 Chapter 2)

Requirements per day: Energy: 2.0 × 100 = 200 kcal ME

Protein: 1.0 × 11.80= 11.80 g CP

Adult cats

Problem 2. Calculate the nutrient requirement of 3 kg active adult cat (three years of age) and formulate a balanced diet.

Metabolic body weight = 2.09 kg

Energy requirement (active cat) =100 kcal ME/kgW$^{0.67}$

(from Table No.10 Chapter 2)

Protein requirement (adults) = 4.96 g/ kgW$^{0.67}$

(from Table No.9 Chapter 2)

Requirements per day: Energy: 2.09 × 100 = 209 kcal ME

Protein: 2.09 × 4.96= 10.37 g CP

Composition of ingredients, per 100 g			1. Balanced kitten diet			2. Balanced cat diet		
Energy, kcal	Protein, g	Ingredient,	Quantity, g	Energy, kcal	Protein, g	Quantity, g	Energy, kcal	Protein, g
67	3.2	Milk	130	87.10	4.16	140	93.80	4.48
194	19	Meat	35	67.90	6.65	25	48.50	4.75
345	6.8	Rice	15	51.75	1.02	20	69.00	1.36
				206.75	11.83		211.30	10.59

Note: Minerals and vitamins supplement need to be provided daily to meet their requirements.

Frequency of Feeding

Dogs should be offered fresh food at least once daily. Free choice feeding could result in excess consumption and weight gain, increasing the risk of developmental bone disease in growing large- and giant-breed dogs and obesity in adults.

Compared to dogs, cats prefer frequent, small meals throughout the day and night. Therefore, dry food offered free-choice is the most practical means of feeding. Again, fresh food should be offered daily to mitigate the risk that spoilage or contamination will hinder normal consumption.

Homemade Diets

Some owners prefer to prepare and feed homemade diets to their pets, while others purchase and feed commercially prepared diets. Preparation of homemade food can be done successfully, if the pet owner is willing to become fully aware of the pet's nutritional requirements, learn the critical aspects of diet formulation, identify and acquire the required ingredients needed for the diet and develop effective processing technology to produce the diet safely on a routine basis. The decision to make homemade pet diets should not be made lightly because the owner is assuming full responsibility for the nutritional status of the pet.

Risks of Some Human Foods Regularly Given to Pets

Common human foods such as raisins, grapes, onions, garlic and chocolate have certain adverse effects when given to dogs or cats either as a treat or leftover from the human food.

Grapes: Gastrointestinal upset followed by acute renal failure. Vomiting, lethargy, anorexia, diarrhoea, abdominal pain, ataxia and weakness are other clinical signs.

Chocolate: Clinical signs start with vomiting, fast heart beating (tachycardia), renal damage, coma and death. Cocoa poisoning was highlighted during the Second World War, when pigs, calves, dogs and horses were poisoned.

Onions and garlic: Regenerative anaemia with marked Heinz body (irreversible oxidative denaturation of haemoglobin) formation has been reported in cats and dogs after eating onions or onion-food (5 to 10 kg/kg BW).

Feeding of Geriatric Dogs and Cats

Guinness records

Today's dogs and cats are living longer. The New Guinness Book of Records 1995 recorded the age of the oldest dog and cat as 29 years and 34 years, respectively.

Geriatric Dog or Cat

The ageing process is influenced by breed size, genetics, nutrition, environment, etc. In general dogs or cats are assigned to 3 life stages: the paediatric stage from birth to 1 year, the maintenance stage from 1 to 8 years and the geriatric stage from 8 years onwards. Some signs of ageing are described as changes in body weight, difficulty in locomotion, changes in hearing and /or eyesight, changes in skin and / or haircoat, changes in urine or bowel habits, and bad breath associated with teeth or mouth problems. Goldston (1989) suggested the following ages to initiate geriatric health care programme in dogs and cats.

> Small dogs (< 9.07 kg): 9 to 13 years
>
> Medium dogs (9.5 – 22.7 kg): 9 to 11.5 years
>
> Large dogs (23.1 – 40.8 kg): 7.5 to 10.5 years
>
> Giant dogs (> 40.8 kg): 6 to 9 years
>
> Cats (most American breeds): 8 to 10 years

Effect of Age on Nutritional Requirements

As a general rule, dogs and cats of 7 years age or older may be considered to be "at risk" for age-related problems. A thorough physical examination should be conducted, including body weight and body condition score, oral examination, skin and hair coat. Increases or decreases in body condition score warrants a detailed dietary history and evaluation since age has a bearing on the nutritional needs (The body condition system (BCS; page no. 63) was developed and tested at the Purina Pet care centre, St. Louis, Missouri, USA)

Energy Needs

The nutritional needs of animals change with their stage of life and their lifestyle or function. Refer tables 3a, b, and c of Chapter 2 for detailed information.

Most commercial foods for geriatric pets contain a reduced concentration of dietary fat and calories. Some foods contain higher dietary fibre to further reduce the caloric density. Monitoring body weight of the geriatric animal is a better guideline in diet allocation rather than assuming that all older pets need reduced calorie intake.

Protein Needs

A classic study was conducted (Wannemacher and McCoy, 1996: J Nutr 88: 66) to determine optimal dietary protein requirements of young and old dogs. The study evaluated the dietary protein needed to maintain nitrogen balance and to maximize liver protein: DNA ratios in 1 to 2 year old Beagles and 12 to 13 year old Beagles. It was found that old dogs actually require up to 50% more protein than young dogs, or at least 3.75 g of protein/kg BW. Similar data for cats are lacking.

PURINA BODY CONDITION SYSTEM

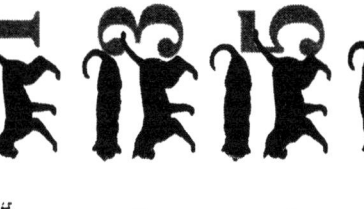
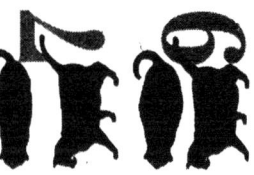
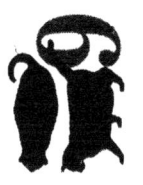

EMACIATED Ribs visible on shorthaired cats; no palpable fat; severe abdominal tuck; lumbar vertebrae and wing of ilia easily palpated.

VERY THIN Shared characteristics of BCS 1 and 3.

THIN Ribs easily palpable with minimal fat covering; lumbar vertebrae obvious; obvious waist behind ribs; minimal abdominal fat.

UNDERWEIGHT Shared characteristics of BCS 3 and 5.

IDEAL Well proportioned; observe waist behind ribs; ribs palpable with slight fat covering; abdominal fat pad minimal.

OVERWEIGHT Shared characteristics of BCS 5 and 7.

HEAVY Ribs not easily palpated with moderate fat covering; waist poorly discernable; obvious rounding of abdomen; moderate abdominal fat pad.

OBESE Shared characteristics of BCS 7 and 9.

GROSSLY OBESE Ribs not palpable under heavy fat cover; heavy fat deposits over lumbar area, face and limbs; distension of abdomen with no waist; extensive abdominal fat deposits.

PURINA BODY CONDITION SYSTEM

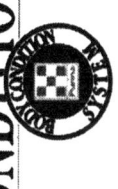
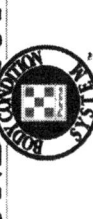

1. **EMACIATED** Ribs, lumbar vertebrae, pelvic bones and all bony prominences evident from a distance. No discernible body fat. Obvious loss of muscle mass.

2. **VERY THIN** Ribs, lumbar vertebrae and pelvic bones easily visible. No palpable fat. Some evidence of other bony prominence. Minimal loss of muscle mass.

3. **THIN** Ribs easily palpated and may be visible with no palpable fat. Tops of lumbar vertebrae visible. Pelvic bones becoming prominent. Obvious waist and abdominal tuck.

4. **UNDERWEIGHT** Ribs easily palpable, with minimal fat covering. Waist easily noted, viewed from above. Abdominal tuck evident.

5. **IDEAL** Ribs palpable without excess fat covering. Waist observed behind ribs when viewed from above. Abdomen tucked up when viewed from side.

6. **OVERWEIGHT** Ribs palpable with slight excess fat covering. Waist is discernable viewed from above but is not prominent. Abdominal tuck apparent.

7. **HEAVY** Ribs palpable with difficulty; heavy fat cover. Noticeable fat deposits over lumbar area and base of tail. Waist absent or barely visible. Abdominal tuck may be absent.

8. **OBESE** Ribs not palpable under very heavy fat cover, or palpable only with significant pressure. Heavy fat deposits over lumbar area and base of tail. Waist absent. No abdominal tuck. Obvious abdominal distention may be present.

9. **GROSSLY OBESE** Massive fat deposits over thorax, spine and base of tail. Waist and abdominal tuck absent. Fat deposits on neck and limbs. Obvious abdominal distension.

It has been suggested that excess dietary protein may cause kidney damage or contribute to the progression of kidney failure. Though the link is logical, studies in dogs and cats have shown that only very high-protein diets (protein content as 38% to 49% of ME) were associated with adverse effects and only in the face of existing renal failure. Moderate - protein diets (up to 34% of diet or 20-31% of energy) had no ill effects and were associated with general improvement as compared with high- or low-(<16% energy)-protein diets.

Other Nutrients

There is currently no published evidence that the requirements for vitamins and minerals differ in healthy, older animals. Patients with subclinical disease associated with a mild malabsorption syndrome or polyuria may have increased loss of water soluble nutrients such as potassium, B-vitamins, or fat soluble vitamins such as vitamins E and A.

Healthy dogs and cats do not experience a significant age-related decline in their ability to digest and absorb nutrients.

Common Nutrient - Sensitive Conditions in Geriatric Animals

Common nutrient-sensitive conditions of older animals include obesity, weight loss, chronic renal failure (CRF) and congestive heart failure (CHF).

Obesity

Approximately 25% of dogs and cats in the United States are overweight or obese. Obesity occurs when a dog repeatedly consumes more energy than he or she expends. In general, a dog whose body weight is 20% or more above the normal weight is considered to be obese. Dogs who are 10% to 15% or more above their ideal body weight should be placed on a weight loss programme. Depending on the degree of obesity and the age and health of the dog, a weight loss of 1% to 2% of the animals total body weight per week is recommended. Weight loss is best accomplished by using a combination of caloric restriction and an exercise programme to increase daily energy expenditure.

As a rule of thumb, an amount of food that provides 60% to 70% of the calories necessary to maintain the dog's current body weight results in adequate weight loss.

Low calorie, high fibre nutritionally balanced diet is suggested for weight loss. Thus, by using these diets, obese pets can receive normal levels of protein and other nutrients while decreasing fat and calorie intake. The fibre in these products may provide a satiety effect.

It is to be noted that gradual weight loss in dogs as in people is more likely to allow long-term maintenance of the reduced body weight. Arthritis is very common in older dogs and cats and it is aggravated by excess body weight. Please refer role of fibre (Page No. 34).

Weight Loss

Weight loss is not unusual in geriatric pets and may be associated with increased or decreased intake. Feed intake is normal or increased but weight loss has been observed. The possible reasons:

- The pet dog should be evaluated for parasitic infestation, pancreatic diseases, renal disease or cancer.
- Malabsorption of nutrients may be involved in such cases; especially fat malabsorption is common in liver and pancreatic diseases and disease involving lymphatic lacteals. In such cases medium chain triglycerides are considered as concentrated source of energy since they are absorbed into portal blood unlike other fats. A high-carbohydrate, low-fat diet is useful in such cases.

Decreased feed intake obviously cause weight loss in geriatric pets. The reasons may be competition among the group of pets in group feeding, poor dental health, appetite loss. Soft foods are the answer for extensive tooth loss.

If no specific cause is found for appetite loss/poor appetite, palatable foods, high-calorie nutrient dense foods are offered to compensate for the less quantity of food intake.

Offer fresh food frequently and encourage the pet to eat more. Chemical appetite stimulants (benzodiazepine, diazepam, oxazepam) may be helpful for short-term use in overcoming anorexia. If adequate intake is not achieved, enteral or parenteral nutritional support should be considered.

Congestive Heart Failure

A thorough nutritional assessment of the geriatric dogs and cats is warranted because certain nutrient sensitive conditions are prevalent in geriatric lifestage. The diet that is offered and feeding management of geriatric animals along with the blood and urine biochemical parameters help the assessment in a holistic way. Accordingly diets have to be recommended considering the client preferences (vegetarian / non-vegetarian) and the food budget of the pets.

Feeding Geriatric Pets

It is important to feed a diet with a lower caloric density (See Tables -3a, b and c in chapter 2) to avoid weight gain, but with a normal protein level to help maintain muscle mass. Studies have shown that the protein requirement for older dogs does not decrease with age, and that protein levels do not contribute to the development or progression of renal failure. It is important to feed older dogs diets that contain optimum levels of highly digestible protein to help in maintaining good muscle mass.

Diets for geriatric animals should contain higher levels of antioxidant nutrients. Antioxidants such as vitamin E and beta-carotene help eliminate free radical particles that can damage body tissues and cause signs of aging. Antioxidants can also increase the effectiveness of the immune system in senior cats and dogs. Antibody response decreases as cats' age, and increasing the intake of vitamin E in cats older than seven years of age can increase their antibody levels back to those seen in younger cats. Gamma-linoleic acid (GLA) is an omega-6 fatty acid that plays a role in the maintenance of healthy skin and coat. Though it is normally produced in a dog's liver, GLA levels may be diminished in older dogs.

Proper nutrition throughout life according to life stage and lifestyle helps ensure that the aging process proceeds as healthily as possible. Such animals have a strong immune system, less- predisposition to becoming ill, and overall healthier and active life compared to those that fed poor quality feed.

Nutritional Diseases

These arise as a direct result of faults in dietary formulation and/or feeding practices.

1. Conditions associated with under-nutrition: e.g. Vitamin or mineral deficiencies; interaction between nutrients - e.g., High levels of Ca in diets may interfere with absorption of other divalent cations such as zinc. High levels of zinc reduce the availability of copper.
2. Conditions associated with overnutrition: e. g. Hypervitaminosis or obesity.

Overnutrition & Skeletal disease: Overnutrition (excessive intake of a food rich in protein, energy, Ca & P) of young, growing puppies (of giant breeds) could result in accelerated growth and a variety of skeletal abnormalities including hypertrophic osteodystrophy, osteochondrosis dissecans and 'wobbler' syndrome. Excessive intake of calcium (diet with 3.3% on DMB) alone could be associated with skeletal changes leading to osteochondrosis, retained cartilage cone, radius curvus syndrome and stunted growth.

Commercial Petfoods (cats and dogs)

Petfood generally falls into dry, semimoist and canned foods categories depending on moisture content.

Dry Petfoods (dry-expanded)

Moisture is 10 to 12%. Most dry foods contain 18 to 27% CP, 7 - 15% fat and 35 to 50% carbohydrate. Ingredients (Table 3) usually present are cereal grains e.g., maize, wheat, oats, barley; cereal grain byproducts e.g., wheat middlings, wheat germ meal, maize gluten meal; soybean products e.g., soybean meal, soy grits; animal byproducts e.g., meat meal, meat and bone meal, meat byproducts, poultry byproducts; milk byproducts e.g., dried skim milk, dried whey; fats and oils e.g., animal fat and micro-and macro-mineral vitamin supplements.

Dry dog foods may be marketed as meal, pellets, kibbles, extruded, or baked products, while dry cat foods are usually processed by extrusion cooking. Cats lack the molar teeth found in dogs. Hence, food particles must be produced for cats in a size and shape suitable for incising rather than grinding by attrition. Extrusion processing is particularly suited for cats (Rokey and Huber, 1994).

The vast majority of dry petfood marketed is extrusion processed. The extrusion process typically results in moderate to high levels of gelatinization of dietary starch. By gelatinizing part or most of the starch, the site of starch hydrolysis (digestion) occurs in the uppergut, resulting in better utilization by the animal with reduced digestive upset.

Table-3. Composition of a dog biscuit

Ingredient	%
Maize	43
Wheat	20
Meat scraps	10
Skim milk powder	10
Soybean meal	5
Groundnut meal	5
Alfalfa meal	2
Bone meal	2
Iodized salt	2
Brewer's yeast	1
	100

Using extrusion processing, a petfood manufacturer can produce a nearly infinite array of shapes, sizes, and colours. This capability is critical in market development but has little to do with the nutritional adequacy of the petfood. After extrusion processing, the injected steam and water used in the process must be removed by drying.

Dry dog and cat foods typically contain 5-12.5 % crude fat, with the majority of the fat being applied post-processing. These fat levels are achieved by spraying a portion of the liquefied fat onto the extruded product. It is also common to spray-coat the petfood with various protein digests and/ or flavours to increase its acceptance by the pet.

Semimoist Petfoods

Moisture is 25 to 30%. Protein normally ranges from 28 to 40% (DM) and crude fat from 10 to 15% (DM). These products are usually cooked through an extrusion process that is very similar to the process used for dry-expanded petfood except the differences in formulations necessary to result in semimoist products. The ingredients used are similar to dry petfood. The meat or meat byproduct slurries are incorporated prior to or during extrusion.

These are protected against spoilage without refrigeration by their content of sucrose, propylene glycol and sorbates. Shelf-life stability is obtained by controlling water activity (amount of free moisture) in the product through these ingredients. Some of these are generally known as "humectants." These bind a large portion of the water and reduce the product's water activity to an acceptable range (<0.60) for shelf stability. It must be noted that propylene glycol is considered "generally recognized as safe" (GRAS) for use in human food products, dog food, and other animal feed (provided specified conditions are met). Federal regulations in USA prohibit the use of propylene glycol in cat food formulations presently.

Semimoist cat foods commonly contain fresh or frozen meats (e.g., liver, kidney), animal byproduct meal (e.g., meat, poultry, liver), whole or dehulled cereal grains (e.g., maize, wheat, rice), marine products (e.g., fish meal, condensed fish solubles), soy products (e.g., soybean meal, soy flour, soy protein concentrate), fats and oils (e.g., animal fat, marine oils), and mineral and vitamin supplements.

Semimoist dog foods are made from similar ingredients but are often shaped into "patties" of a size convenient for feeding or packaged to simulate meat chunks. Semimoist petfoods must be packaged in low-moisture-diffusion packaging to prevent moisture loss and changes in water activity. These foods are commonly marketed in sealed pouches of a size convenient for feeding as a single meal or in a resealable package to control moisture loss.

Soft-expanded (Soft dry) petfoods: It is a category of extrusion processed petfood consisting of soft-expanded petfoods. They often contain a relatively high level of meat byproducts and often have higher levels of fat and oils than dry-expanded foods. Hence, humectants are included to control water activity. They differ from semimoist with respect to taking on an expanded appearance after extrusion. Typical moisture content of soft-expanded petfoods is in the range of 27-32 percent. Soft-expanded foods are often mixed with dry-expanded and semimoist foods to produce a highly palatable food with a texture that is appealing to the pet owner.

Canned Petfoods

The market for canned foods for cats enjoys a sizable market share compared to dog canned foods. Many of the ingredients utilized in canned petfoods are also used in dry-expanded and semimoist petfoods although not at the same level. Canned petfoods are high in moisture, usually 74 to 78%. Hence, they often contain much higher levels of fresh or frozen meat, poultry, or fish products and animal byproducts. A meat-based formulation may contain from 25 to 75% of meat byproducts. Many canned petfoods may contain a significant level of textured protein (either soy- or wheat gluten-based) that is essentially a meat analogue with a structure that mimics the appearance of meat.

Higher energy density dictates higher concentration of protein, vitamins and minerals to overcome nutrient deficiencies. Although these foods are designated to be fed alone as complete and balanced diets, they are commonly used as supplements to improve acceptability of dry foods for feeding during more stressful situations. A variety of petfood diets are available in the market. A summary of the major nutrient content of dry, semimoist, and canned dog food is presented in Table-4. The ranges are similar for the various forms of cat food.

Table-4. Nutrient content of dry, semi-moist, and canned dog foods*

	As-Fed Basis	DM Basis
Dry		
Moisture (%)	6-10	0
Fat (%)	7-20	8-22
Protein (%)	16-30	18-32
Carbohydrate (%)	41-70	46-74

ME (kcal/kg)	2,800-4,050	3,000-4,500
Semimoist		
Moisture (%)	15-30	0
Fat (%)	7-10	8-14
Protein (%)	17-20	20-28
Carbohydrate (%)	40-60	58-72
ME (kcal/kg)	2,550-2,880	3,000-4,000
Canned		
Moisture (%)	75	0
Fat (%)	5-8	20-32
Protein (%)	7-13	28-50
Carbohydrate (%)	4-13	18-57
ME (kcal/kg)	875-1,250	3,500-5,000

*Source: L.P.Case et al. (2000) Types of petfoods pp 187-197 IN: Canine and Feline Nutrition, 2nd Edition, Philadelphia: Mosley

5

Feeding of Sick Animals –
Therapeutic Diets

1. Liver Diseases

Dietary recommendations for dogs vary depending on the underlying cause and severity of liver dysfunction.

For most patients with hepatic dysfunction, the goal for nutritional management is primarily supportive since the patients are at risk for developing malnutrition. Patients are often anorexic, nauseated or vomiting causing decreased food intake. They may have impaired digestion, absorption or metabolism of nutrients. They frequently have increased protein catabolism with reduced protein synthesis. Yet their nutrient requirements are equal or sometimes increased compared to a healthy dog.

It is especially important to ensure that patient has adequate calorie intake. This will not only promote hepatic repair and protein synthesis, but also minimize catabolism of endogenous tissues that generates ammonia. Hence feed a high-carbohydrate diet. Protein plays an important role in hepatic regeneration. Therefore a good amount of protein is required. However, in end stage cirrhosis, protein should be reduced due to hyperammonemia and hepatic encephalopathy.

Increased dietary fibre can benefit patients with hepatobiliary disease in several ways. Dietary fibre reduces the availability and production of nitrogenous wasted in gastrointestinal tract. Increased levels of fermentable fibre increase nitrogen uptake by enteric bacteria. Increased dietary fibre also binds bile acids and endotoxins.

Hypokalemia is a common finding with liver disease due to anorexia, and increased losses through vomiting. Accordingly potassium and sodium, water soluble vitamins and vitamin K are to be supplemented.

71

In dogs without encephalopathy, easily metabolizable starchy and glucose feeds should form the source of energy, and protein of high biological value (animal proteins such as milk, egg) should be fed. A multivitamin preparation should be administered daily. Dietary antioxidants such as vitamins C and E, as well as taurine, may also minimize oxidative damage.

In dogs with hepatic encephalopathy, reduced levels of high-quality protein may be necessary to reduce the accumulation of ammonia and other hepatic toxins. Soluble or moderately fermented fibre helps to reduce the colon pH and absorption of ammonia. In cases of chronic liver diseases and ascites, feeding of high sodium feeds and common salt are restricted / avoided.

Feline hepatic lipidosis: It usually occurs in obese cats. The affected ones may be anorectic. Most cats will require a feeding tube. Energy-dense, high-protein diets are usually selected for cats without encephalopathy. The increase of energy and protein need to be introduced gradually to prevent complications, such as vomiting or electrolyte abnormalities. Carnitine supplementation is also beneficial in cats with hepatic lipidosis. Fluid needs must be met and parenteral fluid support may be needed in many cats. In cats with encephalopathy, dietary protein may need to be restricted.

2. Diabetes Mellitus (DM)

It is a chronic endocrine disorder caused by the relative or absolute deficiency of the hormone insulin. Hence there is no blood glucose homeostasis. The most common form of DM in dogs is insulin-dependent DM, or Type I diabetes, which occurs when the pancreas is incapable of producing or secreting insulin. Non-insulin dependent DM or Type II diabetes occurs when there is a relative deficiency of insulin. Insulin injections may be needed to control hyperglycemia. Owners usually first notice an increase in water consumption (polydypsia), an increase in urination (polyuria) and occasionally weight loss.

- Complex carbohydrates should make up more than 40% of the calories because digestion of complex carbohydrates provides glucose to the blood stream at a slower rate than simple carbohydrates.
- Fat should be moderately restricted to 18 to 20% of calories.
- Dietary protein should be of high quality and included in quantities that meet but do not greatly exceed the dog's requirement.
- A dry-type dog food formulated for maintenance or for less active adults is appropriate for diabetic pets.
- Portion-controlled meal feeding should be used (several small meals)
- Green vegetables, bran-enriched chapatti, skim milk should be included. (Also see glycemic response of diet, page No 35).

Cats most commonly develop type II DM, although some cats may develop type I often secondary to chronic pancreatitis. The most common risk factors for DM in cats are obesity and increasing age. Feline DM is similar to type II DM in people. Feeding diabetic cats a diet high in protein (more than 45 % of calories) and low in carbohydrates (less than 20 % of calories) improves glucose regulation.

3. Diarrhoea

Diarrhoea can result from numerous GI diseases and can also occur secondary to disease outside the GI tract. Clinical signs associated with diarrhoea are different and vary with the section of the intestine affected. Dietary recommendations may vary depending on where the diarrhoea is localized and the underlying cause.

Animals with small-bowel diarrhoea usually benefit from a highly digestible diet, while those with large-bowel diarrhoea often benefit from prebiotics. Small, frequent meals (3-6/ day) should be offered. Probiotics are an additional tool available for management of small- or large-bowel diarrhoea. Synbiotics are a mixture of prebiotics and probiotics in which the prebiotic increases the survival of and nourishes the probiotic bacteria.

The diet should contain low fibre cereals, low protein and easily digestible protein foods like paneer, cottage-cheese, curd, eggs and liver. It should not contain more than 10-12 per cent fat on dry matter basis. A high paneer or high egg diet should be supplemented for potassium deficiency. Oral rehydration therapy (giving plenty of fluids rich in electrolytes) is important. In acute case parenteral fluid feeding may be necessary to restore the body fluid volume and electrolytes. The following soft liquid diet (Table 1) may be useful to feed sick animals.

Table 1:   Composition of a soft liquid diet

Food ingredient	Quantity
Cooked rice gruel or low fibre wheat flour gruel or sago gruel (100g DM)	500 ml
Sugar	60 g
Paneer or Cottage-cheese (50 g DM)	200 g
Cream (30 g DM)	100 g
Maize-oil or safflower-oil	15 g
Hard cooked egg	100 g
Dicalcium phosphate	10 g
Potassium chloride	15 g
Mineral vitamin supplement	as per the dose on the container

Note: The above diet should be fed @ 100 ml per kg body weight daily in 5-6 split meals at equal interval

4. Gastroenteritis

Bland diets (high quality, highly digestible and non-spicy diet) are to be fed when a dog is suffering from gastroenteritis. The diet may be prepared from chicken soup, egg white, milk, sago, vegetable soup, sugar and cream supplemented with dicalcium phosphate, trace minerals and vitamins.

5. Pyrexia (fever)

Energy requirement of dog increases in fever. High energy bland diet using cream, egg or maize oil is offered to such animal. In case of anorexia, fluid diet should be administered with the help of a stomach tube.

6. Vomiting

Vomiting may be due to eating of spoiled foods or disease. Normally feeding should be avoided for the day. The sick animals should be offered fresh light diet as suggested for diarrhoea.

7. Stress Conditions

Dogs exposed to hostile environmental conditions like extreme cold or heat should be provided a high energy food at short intervals of 2-4 hours depending on the severity of exposure. A 50 per cent glucose solution @ 70 ml per kg body weight should be given orally in split meals at 3 hours intervals and the animal should be offered fresh drinking water about 40-50 ml per kg body weight during the first 24 hours. Table sugar solution can be administered in the absence of glucose or fructose. In case of sunstroke parenteral fluid therapy may be essential.

8. Urolithiasis

Low protein, low mineral food containing high percentage of common salt should be fed to increase water intake and urine volume. An increase in urination frequency and urine volume reduces the chances to form uroliths. In case the composition of uroliths is known (oxalates, etc) special diets low in such substances need to be formulated.

9. Urinary Calculi in Cats

Most (90-97%) of the urinary calculi in cats with Feline Urologic Syndrome (FUS) are composed exclusively or primarily of struvite (magnesium-ammonium-phosphate). It may also be referred to as Feline lower urinary tract disease (FLUTD). Feline urine always contains high amounts of ammonium due to cat's high protein requirement and intake. Urinary phosphate in the normal healthy cat is also high enough for struvite formation, regardless of dietary P intake.

The concentration of urinary Mg is normally quite low and can be directly affected by the level of dietary intake. Magnesium is widespread in foods, especially of vegetable origin. High dietary intakes of magnesium have been linked with an increased risk of FLUTD due to an increase in the risk of struvite formation. Struvite is more soluble in acid than in alkaline medium.

Struvite calculi will form in feline urine with a pH of 7.0 or greater, and its solubility greatly increases at a pH of 6.6 or less. Compared to an omnivorous or herbivorous diet, a true carnivorous diet has the effect of increasing net acid excretion and decreasing urinary pH. This urinary acidifying effect is due primarily to the high level of S-containing amino acids in meats. The oxidation of amino acids results in the excretion of sulfate in the urine and a concomitant decrease in urinary pH.

A high meat diet is lower in K salts than is a diet containing high amounts of cereal grains (High cereal grain diet produce alkaline urine). The inclusion of high amount of cereal grains and low amount of meat products may be a contributing factor to the development of FUS in cats.

Hypokalaemic polymyopathy: It has been observed in cats under specific circumstances. Inclusion of dietary potassium above 0.5% is suggested in diets designed for urinary acidification or for cats with renal failure.

10. Chronic Kidney Disease

The kidney has many regulatory and excretory functions and is essential for normal homeostasis and health. The functional units of the kidney are called nephrons. The kidney has a significant reserve capacity and ability to compensate for damage or disease. As a result, clinical signs of kidney disease will be observed only after a loss of 70 to 85% of functioning nephrons has occurred. Chronic renal failure (CRF) occurs over weeks to years in contrast to acute renal failure that occurs within hours or days. The animal is unable to eliminate the waste products of protein metabolism.

Signs and symptoms: One of the first signs owners notice in the dog is increased water consumption and increased urination. Azotemia (accumulation of nitrogenous waste products such as creatinine in the blood) and uremia (elevated concentration of urea in the blood); decreased appetite, vomiting, electrolyte and pH disturbances are also observed. Calcium and phosphorus homeostasis are negatively affected in dogs with renal disease. Overtime, these changes lead to bone demineralization. The inability of the kidney to produce the hormone erythropoietin, which is necessary for the production of red blood cells, can lead to anaemia in some dogs.

Elevated plasma levels of urea and other waste products cause nausea, vomiting and anorexia. Enticing them to eat is a major challenge of dietary therapy. Glucose may be fed to anorectic dogs to prevent catabolism of protein and to supply energy. Fat addition in the diet makes the diet more palatable and may stimulate increased consumption in sick pets. Adequate water supply should be made to encourage urination. Sometimes little salt may be provided (if the dog has no cardiac problem) as it acts as saline diuretic.

The phosphorus content of diet is important because dogs with chronic kidney disease have a decreased ability to excrete this mineral. Dietary restriction of phosphorus is helpful in the early stages of renal diseases. In more severe cases, phosphate binding agents such as aluminium hydroxide and aluminium carbonate must be used in conjunction with reduced dietary phosphorus to normalize serum phosphorus concentration.

Nutritional management of chronic kidney disease

(i) The objective of dietary management in renal failure is to lessen the metabolic demands on the kidneys and to diminish metabolic end-products that cannot be readily excreted. Energy should be supplied primarily via feeding relatively more digestible fat and carbohydrates.

(ii) Restrict dietary protein when there are clinical signs of uremia and blood urea nitrogen (BUN) is greater than 60 mg/dl.

(iii) A diet that contains high quality protein and adequate levels of nonprotein calories from fat and carbohydrate should be selected.

(iv) Diets with protein restriction to 20-31% ME or 12-16% ME (depending on the clinical symptoms) or straight forwardly 2g protein/kg BW and phosphorus restriction to less than 0.4% of dry matter should be used in dogs with chronic renal failure. Calcium carbonate / calcium lactate is used to bind the intestinal phosphorus if needed to control the phosphorus level in blood.

(v) Adjustments in dietary sodium may be necessary if secondary hypertension develops.

(vi) Provide supplemental water soluble vitamins if polyuria leads to excessive losses.

(vii) In cats the dietary management is complicated by hypokalemia and potassium deficiency may cause as well as be caused by CRF.

(viii) Cats with CRF also appear to benefit from a phosphorus restricted diet. However, cats fed protein restricted diets (28% CP) should be monitored carefully to assure adequate protein intake.

 (ix) Oral supplementation of potassium (as potassium gluconate) may stabilize or even reverse renal dysfunction and this supplementation may be continued based on serum potassium concentration.

  (x) Diets with at least 0.7% potassium (dry matter basis) without a dietary acidifier (such as those intended for the prevention of struvite urolithiasis) are suggested for such cats because inadequate potassium intake and dietary acidification have been implicated as contributing factors.

11. Congestive Heart Failure (CHF)

One objective in managing congestive heart failure (CHF) is to reduce water retention. Restricting sodium intake and lowering sodium levels encourage diuresis. Dietary sodium restriction is classified as mild (400 mg sodium/100 g diet) to severe (240 mg sodium/100 g diet DM). Although dietary sodium restriction is given priority, energy intake and specific nutrients such as potassium, magnesium and taurine are of particular concern.

Carnitine is also an essential nutrient in some breeds of dogs (Boxers, American Cocker Spaniel) with myocardial disease.

Taurine is recognized as an essential nutrient in the cat but not the dog. Most commercial cat foods are fortified with additional taurine because of the clinical association between plasma taurine deficiency and dilated cardiomyopathy (DCM).

In cardiac patients hepatic congestion, portal hypertension, pulmonary congestion may occur which lead to decreased gastrointestinal function and respiratory acidosis.

Pulmonary congestion increases the work of breathing, greatly increasing the energy spent for this purpose. Severe congestion and dyspnea also contributes to anorexia. Diuretics induce the loss of potassium, magnesium, calcium and B-vitamins.

Anorexia coupled with decreased gastrointestinal function (that is decreased ability to digest and absorb nutrients), urinary loss of nutrients, and greater energy expenditure may contribute to cardiac cachexia which causes additional risks for patients with heart disease.

Calorie intake of the cardiac patients with either obesity or cachexia needs to be monitored closely. Obesity should be controlled to reduce the workload on the heart. Highly digestible, high-calorie diets should be offered several times in a day to cachectic patients to help enhance calorie absorption. Diets should have surplus amounts of B-vitamins and minerals to compensate for losses induced by diuretics. Patients with CHF should not be fed acidifying diets because of likelihood of acidosis in CHF and the link between acidifying diets and depletion of both taurine and potassium.

Oral supplementation of taurine (one gram per day) and L-Carnitine (two grams per day) are quite beneficial in certain breeds of dogs with cardiomyopathy.

12. Anaemia

Iron or copper deficiency is the major cause of hypochromic, microcytic anaemia. A folic acid and B_{12} deficiency also produces anaemia. Most commercial diets have more than the required amount of iron, copper and vitamins. Secondary causes such as haemorrhage, heavy parasitism need to be looked into; inadequate food intake, malabsorption may also be kept in mind. Feeding imbalanced homemade food also causes anaemia.

Severe iron deficiency may not be corrected with diet alone. Feeding large quantities of liver in an attempt to correct iron deficiency can result in vitamin A toxicosis. Most animals require a supplemental source of iron administered via intramuscular route to correct the deficiency.

Folic acid and vitamin B_{12} are necessary to support normal cell division, and treatment of vitamin B_{12} deficiency usually requires parenteral administration of vitamin B_{12}. Vitamin B_{12} deficiency develops most commonly from intestinal malabsorption. Since the absorption of B_{12} vitamin is limited to the ileum, surgical removal of large portions of the ileum may result in the need for lifelong parenteral B_{12} supplementation.

13. Metabolic Syndrome

The metabolic syndrome was developed as a pathophysiological entity in humans after it was highlighted by Reaven (1988), who argued that insulin resistance was the pathophysiological driver of the metabolic syndrome, type 2 diabetes and cardiovascular disease (Reaven, 2011). Metabolic syndrome is a condition of at least three of the cardiovascular risk factors: obesity, excessive visceral fat storage, dyslipidemia, hypertension and hyperglycaemia or Type 2 diabetes. A recent consensus statement harmonized the definition of the metabolic syndrome as the presence of 3/5 components: plasma triglyceride > 150 mg/dl; HDL cholesterol < 40 mg/dl in men or 50 mg/dl in women; blood pressure > 135/85 mmHg; plasma glucose > 100 mg/dl and gender- and ethnicity-adjusted excessive waist circumference (Albert et al., 2006, 2009).

The human metabolic syndrome: The metabolic syndrome in humans causes neither clinical signs nor mortality. Its importance is that it is a useful pathophysiological concept. The components of the metabolic syndrome are worth treating in humans because each is an independent risk factor for clinical disease and mortality and the consequences of the metabolic syndrome in humans give validity to the metabolic syndrome.

The metabolic syndrome in dogs: There are two ways of looking at the metabolic syndrome, as a set of components, or as a set of consequences. Dogs develop many of the components of the metabolic syndrome: obesity, insulin resistance, increased blood pressure and hyperlipidaemia. Unlike humans, however, obese dogs do not develop fasting hyperglycaemia or atherogenic hyperlipidaemia. Importantly, there is no evidence that dogs develop type 2 diabetes. Atherosclerosis, coronary heart disease and stroke are rare and not known to be associated with obesity in dogs. On the basis of current knowledge, Verkset (2013) opines that the use of the term 'metabolic syndrome' in dogs does not appear to have merit.

Foods for Specific Dietary Purposes (e.g., Medical foods)

Use of laboratory dogs or cats as models for certain animal or human diseases makes the necessity to modify the nutrient composition of the diet to feed them.

Lower levels of protein and phosphorus in diets intended for animals with compromised renal function may help mitigate clinical manifestations of the disease and provide for a more normal quality of life (Allen et al., 2000). Similar restrictions on other nutrient components may ameliorate signs of other disease processes, such as sodium in cardiac insufficiency and copper in breed-associated liver storage disease. This only reiterates that lowering these levels closer to the minimum requirements helps alleviate signs of disease; it should not in most cases compromise nutritional adequacy.

Commercial diets intended for medical use are held to the same nutritional standards as any other dog or cat foods (AAFCO, 2003).

Special considerations also apply to the postoperative laboratory animal. Feeding these animals may necessitate use of a more palatable and/or nutrient-dense food to encourage adequate consumption. Inadequate intake of nutrients can affect both immunocompetence and tissue repair, compromising surgical recovery. Also, trauma from the procedure may result in catabolic state, which could at least be ameliorated partially by increased energy and other nutrient intakes.

In extreme conditions of anorexia or where the procedure itself limits voluntary consumption, use of a balanced liquid or gel form 'dog or cat product' can be delivered by a feeding tube. Although the gastrointestinal tract is always the preferred route of administration, parenteral nutrition may be necessary on a temporary basis when the surgery or other experimental procedure compromises gut function.

Malabsorption Syndrome

The animal's gastrointestinal tract (GIT) is an interface with the environment. GIT is the last line of defence against the entry of pathogens into the body proper. Feed consumption continually exposes the GIT to feed ingredients, toxins and microorganisms which may damage the structure and have serious health consequences. This leads to malabsorption of nutrients, diarrhoea, etc.

The term 'malabsorption syndrome' is used to describe a number of disorders that are characterized by steatorrhoea and multiple abnormalities in absorption of nutrients.

Malabsorption in these disorders may be due to defects in the intenstinal lumen, resulting in inadequate fat hydrolysis or altered bile salt metabolism. Inadequate production of lipase occurs in pancreatic insufficiency and inadequate amounts of conjugated bile salts due to hepatobiliary disease, etc.

Malabsorption in these disorders may also be due to defects in the mucosal epithelial cells, affecting absorbing surfaces and interfering with transport functions; absence or deficiency of specific enzymes or failure of proper regulation of enzyme activity in the cell interferes with the absorption of certain nutrients and produces symptoms of malabsorption or intestinal lymphatics.

Dietary Modification

Generally speaking, the diet in malabsorption syndrome should be high in protein and calories. In certain disorders elimination of specific carbohydrates or proteins is necessary. Modification of fat is often indicated. Vitamin and mineral supplementation is usually needed. A soft or fibre-restricted diet is useful for patients with persistent diarrhoea.

Fat absorption can be improved in some malabsorptive disorders by changing the type of fat ingested. Medium-chain triglycerides (MCT) (fatty acids with 8 to 10 carbon atoms) are hydrolyzed much more rapidly than long-chain fats (LCT) in the intestinal lumen. The presence of pancreatic enzymes and bile salts are not required for absorption of the fats of medium-chain length. MCT are transported by way of the portal vein as free fatty acids bound to albumin whereas long-chain fats must undergo esterification and chylomicron formation and are transported by way of the lymph.

Lactase Deficiency

In the absence of lactase, lactose is not hydrolyzed to glucose and galactose. The accumulation of lactose in the intestine causes fermentation, abdominal pain, cramping and diarrhoea. Lactose-free diet is the remedy.

Sucrase-isomaltase Deficiency

Deficiency of these enzymes lead to symptoms similar to those seen in lactase insufficiency following ingestion of significant amounts of sucrose and isomaltose. Wheat and potato starches should be avoided as these yield more isomaltose upon hydrolysis than do other starches such as rice and maize.

Glucose-galactose Deficiency

This rare disease is characterized by inability to absorb any carbohydrate that yields glucose or galactose upon hydrolysis.

Adverse Reaction to Foods

Adverse reaction to foods can be of two types as food intolerance and food allergy. (1) Food intolerance is a type of adverse reaction that does not involve the immune system, e.g. food poisoning. (2) A food allergy is a type of adverse reaction that does involve the immune system, e.g. colitis or atopic dermatitis. Dogs and cats with food allergy usually have gastrointestinal signs or a pruritic skin condition.

Therapeutic diets / Modified diets

Nutrition is an important part of disease management, even though few disorders can be cured solely with diet. Optimal nutrition is essential for normal growth and the maintenance of health and vitality throughout life. Supplementation, overfeeding, or providing inappropriate items can lead to nutritional disorders or illness. Several health problems in dogs can be treated or managed through diet. Dietary therapy often plays an important role.

The purposes of diet therapy are to maintain good nutritional status, correct the deficiencies that may have occurred, afford rest to the whole body or to certain organs that may be affected, adjust the food intake to the body's ability to metabolize the nutrients and bring about changes in body weight whenever necessary.

Diet therapy deals with modifications necessary in the diet in the treatment of different diseases. This is necessary as the metabolism of the individual changes in different diseases with respect to one or more nutrients.

Examples: Inefficient utilization of carbohydrates in diabetes mellitus, inability of the kidney to excrete sodium chloride in nephritis, increased production and inefficient elimination of uric acid in gout and increase in energy metabolism and in the catabolism of tissue protein in fever.

The simplest modification of diets is in the treatment of allergy where the food or foods responsible for the allergic reactions are eliminated. The other modifications include modifying the nutrient level and consistency of the diet. These are

1. Bland diets omitting condiments and spices
2. Low fibre or high fibre diets
3. High protein or low protein diets
4. High fat or low fat diets
5. High carbohydrate or low carbohydrate diets
6. High calorie or low calorie diets
7. Low sodium diets and
8. Low purine diets.

Modifications in Carbohydrate Content

High carbohydrate diet may be indicated in Addison's disease (Adrenal cortex insufficiency), various diseases of the liver and in the pre-operative conditions.

Restricted carbohydrate diet is essential in the treatment of diabetes mellitus. See Appendix for Addison's disease and Cushing's disease.

Modifications in Calorie Content

Diets with increased calorie value are used for the treatment of patients who are markedly underweight, and also for patients with increased calorie requirements as in fever, infections, malabsorption and hyperthyroidism.

Low calorie diets are used for the treatment of obesity, cardiovascular disease, acute uraemia and hepatic coma.

Modifications in Protein Content

High protein diets (i.e. about twice the actual requirements) with restriction in other nutrients are prescribed in a variety of diseases such as protein-calorie malnutrition, cirrhosis of liver, peptic ulcer, nephrosis and celiac diseases.

Low protein or complete withdrawal of protein may be necessary in hepatic coma, acute uraemia, etc.

Modifications in Fat Content

Moderately high fat diet is used in the treatment of severe under nutrition. Restricted or low fat diet may be necessary in the treatment of steatorrhoea, malabsorption syndrome and diseases of the liver.

Modifications in Mineral Content

High calcium diet is essential in the treatment of rickets and osteomalacia, while a diet restricted in calcium and phosphate is desirable in renal calculi. Sodium restricted diets are essential in the treatment of cardiac failure and hypertension. Restriction in salt intake is essential in diseases of kidneys.

Modifications in Vitamin Content

Increase in the content of vitamins can be easily achieved by the addition of synthetic vitamins. This is essential as most of the therapeutic diets may be partially lacking in one or more vitamins.

Modifications in Fibre Content

Diets rich in fibre are prescribed for the treatment of constipation, while low-fibre diets are essential in the treatment of several gastrointestinal disorders such as peptic ulcer, ulcerative colitis, celiac diseases, diarrhoea and dysentery. See Appendix for Celiac disease in canines.

Modifications in Other Constituents

Diets low in purine content is prescribed in treatment of gout. Gout is considered as hereditary disease resulting from defective uric acid metabolism. Serum uric acid levels are raised and urates (sodium salt of uric acid) are deposited in the cartilage and articular cartilage of the joints. There are recurrent attacks of pain and swelling of the joints. Diets low in oxalic acid and purines are prescribed in renal calculi.

Oral and Intravenous Feeds for Sick Animals

Oral Feeding and Nasogastric Feeding

The most important are the liquid diets used in oral feeding and nasogastric feeding. Here the diet consistency is modified. The basis of such diets is milk to which soluble carbohydrates such as sucrose, glucose and dextrimaltose and emulsified fats are added to increase their calorific value. These include (1) Clear-fluid diets (2) Full-fluid diets and (3) Soft Diets.

1. Clear-Fluid Diets

Clear-fluid diets are prescribed for patients with marked intolerance to foods as manifested by nausea, vomiting, loss of appetite etc. These are usually used for 1 or 2 days and are meant to provide some calories and make-up the water loss in the body e.g. Glucose water (10%), Barley water (with glucose), Tender coconut water, Orange juice.

2. Full-fluid Diets:

Full-fluid diets are prescribed when the patient (human) is unable to chew or swallow solid foods.

Table 1. Composition of Full-fluid Diet (per day)

Foodstuff	Veg.	Non-Veg.
Corn flour, g	50	50
Dhal flour, g	30	--
Milk, ml	1000	800
Meat, g	–	50
Egg	–	one
Fruit juice, ml	800	800
Butter, g	60	60
Sugar, g	100	100

3. Soft Diets

Soft diets are used in acute infection, gastrointestinal disorder and in post-operative cases.

Serious malabsorption of nutrients may occur especially in liver diseases and those involving the gastrointestinal tract. Extensive losses of nutrients and fluids may have occurred through haemorrhage, vomiting, or diarrhoea.

Table 2. Composition of Soft Diet (g/caput/day) for human patient

Foodstuff	Veg.	Non-Veg.
Rice (345 kcal/kg; 6.8% CP)	300	300
Bread (244 kcal/kg; 8.8% CP)		
Green gram dhal	50	30
(348 kcal/kg; 24.5% CP)		
Milk (67; 3.2)	1000	600
Meat and fish (196, 126; 18.2, 22.5)	–	100
Egg (146, 11.3)	–	One
Cheese (348; 24.1)	80	30
Vegetables (Beans, 49; 4.70)	50	50
Potato (97; 1.6)	100	100
GLV (50; 4.5)	100	100
Orange fruits (48; 0.7)	100	100
Butter and oils (900; -)	30	30
Sugar (400; -)	80	80

Following surgery or injury the need for nutrients is greatly increased as a result of loss of blood, plasma, or pus from the wound surface; haemorrhage from the gastrointestinal or pulmonary tract; vomiting and fever. During immobilization, the loss of some nutrients such as protein is accelerated.

Enteral Nutrition

Enterals are sterile liquid nutritionally complete dietary products manufactured primarily for hospitalised humans. Used commonly in critically-ill patients. Enteral nutrition has been proved to be physiological and better tolerated than parenteral nutrition in terms of cost, ease of administration and associated complications. Nowadays readymade enteral diets are available. Use of such readymade enteral diets improve the overall nutritional status, diminish morbidity and reduce the duration of hospitalisation and induce anabolism in patients suffering from cancer, burns or other catabolic conditions.

Glutamine Enriched Enteral Nutrition

Glutamine is a non-essential amino acid widely distributed throughout the body. It can behave as an essential amino acid in certain clinical settings. Glutamine improves immunologic function by decreasing the inflammatory response and infectious morbidity in patients with multiple traumas.

Emerging application of n-3 fatty acids in surgical or critically-ill patients

Excessive or inappropriate inflammation and immunosuppression are components of the response to surgery, trauma, injury and infection in some individuals and these can lead, progressively, to sepsis and septic shock (P.C.Calder, 2010). N-3 fatty acids from fish oil decrease the production of inflammatory cytokines and eicosanoids. They act both directly (by replacing arachidonic acid as an eicosanoid precursor) and indirectly (by altering the expression of inflammatory genes through effects on transcription factor activation).

Total Parenteral Nutrition (TPN)

Total parenteral nutrition (TPN) is a potent pharmacologic therapy that feeds nutrients, electrolytes, trace minerals, vitamins, and medications directly into the bloodstream. Parenteral nutrition support is necessary in a large group of severely injured trauma patients, and many critically-ill patients in the intensive care unit. Some patients with gastrointestinal problems cannot be fed enterally, and it is necessary to maintain their nutrient intake with parenteral nutrition.

The main objectives in intravenous feeding are: (1) to provide water and electrolytes to prevent dehydration and correct electrolyte imbalance, (2) to make up the loss of tissue proteins and (3) to provide energy to meet the daily needs of the patients.

The concept of feeding patients entirely parenterally (total parenteral nutrition, TPN) by injecting nutrient substances or fluids intravenously was advocated four decades ago. Most clinicians in the 1950's were aware of the negative impact of starvation on morbidity, mortality, and outcomes, but only few understood the necessity for providing adequate nutritional support to malnourished patients if optimal clinical results were to be achieved (S.J.Dudrick, 2009). **The prevailing dogma in the 1960's was that, "Feeding entirely by vein is impossible; even if it were possible, it would be impractical; and even if it were practical, it would be unaffordable."**

Prescribing TPN: Here human patient is used as an example. The amount of TPN given is usually determined by first calculating the protein requirement (1.5 - 2g/kg /day). Then adequate carbohydrate is provided (150 Kcal/g N_2) to allow use of carbohydrate catabolism to support protein anabolism (70% of daily non-protein needs are through carbohydrates). Fat, electrolytes, vitamins, and mineral elements (Na, K, Mg, Ca, phosphates, chlorides and acetate; Zn, Cu, Cr, Se and Mn) are then added to complete the prescription. Lipids are included to provide up to 30% of a patient's daily caloric requirements. Lipid emulsions are available in 10% (1 Kcal/mL) and 20% (2 Kcal/mL) strengths. Non-protein caloric requirement = 25 Kcal/kg/day. After starting the therapy, appropriate laboratory studies (serum glucose, electrolyte levels and liver function tests) are performed to monitor the patient's physiologic state. In addition to these supplements, a TPN recipient must receive a 5 to 10 mg intramuscular dose of vitamin K on a weekly basis.

For severely debilitated patients, TPN is useful in providing complete nutritional support for extended periods. The method involves passage of an indwelling catheter into the superiorvena cava with continous infusion of a hypertonic solution of 20 to 25% glucose, 3 to 5% protein hydrolysate or amino acids, vitamins and minerals. Linoleic acid is also added. A minimum of 8g N_2 and 1800 Kcal energy daily are required for positive N balance. Intravenous fat emulsions make possible a substantial increase in caloric intake and promote positive N balance.

The nutrients used in 'nutshell' are

1. Water and electrolytes e.g. normal saline
2. Carbohydrates and alcohol e.g. 5% dextrose, 3% alcohol (Alcohol provides 7.1 Kcal/g)
3. Amino acids e.g. 3% amino acid solution with electrolytes.
4. Whole blood or plasma
5. Emulsified fat and
6. Vitamins

The most important complication of parenteral nutrition is sepsis. An antibiotic - antifungal cream should be placed at the catheter insertion site.

PART II
Wild Animal Nutrition

6

Nutrition Research of Wild Animals and Birds

Wildlife

According to Wildlife Protection Act, "wildlife" is defined as 'any animal, bee, butterflies, crustaceae, fish and moths and aquatic or land vegetation'. Thus it is to be understood that wildlife is the term that embraces all life forms that are wild or care themselves.

Nutrition of Wildlife

Knowledge of wildlife nutrition is central to understanding the survival and productivity of all wildlife populations, whether free-ranging or captive. The science of wildlife nutrition is an extremely young area of investigation. It all began during the early 1880s when ornithologists and entomologists started investigating the food habits of wildlife in relation to the welfare of humans (W.L.McAtee, 1933). The number of wildlife nutrition studies has increased markedly since 1937, and particularly since 1960. This post-1960 surge presumably reflects the increased interest in the broad areas of animal biology, the environment and ecology. The increasing number of studies, especially in 1990s, is indicative of a growing body of information relative to all aspects of wildlife nutrition. Dr.Charles T.Robbins did an excellent job in compiling an enormous amount of information on wildlife nutrition in the 2nd edition of "Wildlife Feeding and Nutrition" 1993.

Nutrition of Captive and Free-ranging Wildlife

Nondomesticated and nonlaboratory species are not dealt in standard Animal Nutrition courses and thus in standard Animal Nutrition Textbooks. There is a felt need for information on captive animal nutrition, feed resources and nutrition of free-ranging wildlife. Feeding and nutrition of free-ranging wildlife is much more complex than the feeding of farm livestock and poultry (Charles T.Robbins, 1993). The wildlife nutritionist often does have much more of a comparative perspective than does the domestic animal nutritionist.

Nutrition Research of Wildlife Species vis-à-vis Domestic Animals

Nutrition research and management of wildlife species offer many challenges not always encountered by the scientist working with domestic animals. These are primarily because of the need to maintain an ecological perspective in designing and implementing any wildlife nutrition research (A.Watson, 1973). The free-ranging animal is constantly changing environment, and humans have little control over many of the animal-environment interactions. The lack of control over wild free-ranging animals often requires that the wildlife ecologists need to have a greater base of knowledge to understand such interactions than the scientist working with domestic animals. Nutrition studies conducted in such ecological systems generate results which are often essential to understanding other living systems.

Nutritionist working with domestic animals aims for maximizing milk/ meat production or economic return, while the wildlife ecologist/nutritionist looks for conservation and control of wildlife populations. The wildlife nutritionist need not consider catabolism and weight loss as undesirable. It is considered as essential components of life strategies of many wild animals. Many captive wild animals have seasonal gain-loss cycles even in the presence of abundant food. This indicates the importance of weight loss.

Wild Animal Nutrition - an Emerging Discipline

With the passage of time life style of mankind has changed greatly. Tendency of show, ego and exhibition of socio-economical superiority in the society took upper hand. The advent of newer technologies increased the easy availability of human amenities. Newer technologies and the craze for items of luxury resulted in the devastating depletion of some of the natural resources. One of the highly depleted natural resources is forest and thus the forest dependent resources including the wildlife. Shrinkage in the area of forests has reduced the availability of feedstuffs and shelter causing reduction in the population of wild animals. Several species became extinct and many are endangered. Man-animal conflicts are happening frequently in the forest-adjoining areas.

Endangered species require special protection for which arrangements have been made in captive conditions of zoological parks and national parks of reserved forests. The changes in habitat from free-ranging to captive conditions require research studies to know their nutrient requirements, method of feeding and feeding behaviour and the skill of feeding management. American Association of Zoos and Aquariums recognized the importance of nutrition as a scientific specialty for the proper management of zoo animals (Dierenfeld, 1997). In IVRI, Izatnagar (India), N.N.Pathak, D.N.Kamra and coworkers initiated studies in 1990s in blackbuck (*Antilope cervicapra*) and hog deer (*Axis porcinus*) on their feeding in captive environment.

The Centre of Advanced Studies (presently known as Centre of Advanced Faculty Training) in Animal Nutrition, since its inception in 1995 (IVRI, Izatnagar, India) with its Directors Drs S.P.S.Bedi, N.N.Pathak, D.K.Agarwal, Usha Rani Mehra, Kusumakar Sharma, D.N.Kamra and R.S.Dass, contributed greatly to the scientific knowledge and human resource development in animal nutrition in the country. Specially short courses on 'Nutrition and Feeding of Wild and Zoo animals' had been conducted by Dr N.N.Pathak (in 1996), Dr D.K.Agarwal (in 2000) and Dr K.Sharma (in 2008) and a short course on 'Clinical Nutrition of Livestock and Pet animals' was conducted by Dr K.Sharma (in 2006) to train the scientists and teachers in feeding management of pet and wild animals.

7

Zoos - Control and Conservation of Wildlife - Food chain

Zoo is a place wherein the collection and breeding of wild animals including birds are carried out in a systematic manner in captivity.

Primary Goal of Zoos

1. **The primary goal of zoos was entertainment during earlier times.** Our knowledge of captive animals is not much though we have a long history of zoos. It is reported that 60-70% of the animals died in zoos prior to 1970 because of poor management and husbandry, with 25% died due to nutritional problems (Wallach, 1970).

2. **Conservation and propagation of rare species:** Now the major goal of zoos is conservation (Table 1) and propagation of rare species apart from creating awareness of them, which is also a source of entertainment.

3. **The mandate of the zoos** (or rather it is emphasized) is to have healthy and reproducing animals and thus the zoo animals are to be fed nutritious and palatable diets. There is a need to understand the nutritional needs of each species.

4. **Zoos are a valuable resource to the development of wildlife nutrition** because of the availability of variety of (captive) species in zoos and the unique facilities available there.

Ectotherm: Ectotherms are also called cold-blooded animals, i.e., any animal whose regulation of body temperature depends on external sources, such as sunlight or a heated rock surface. The ectotherms include the fishes, amphibians, reptiles, and invertebrates. The body temperatures of aquatic

Table 1. **General groups of animals that are managed for control or conservation of populations***

Taxa	Group	Energy demand	Trophic level	Typical application**
Fish	Marine: reef fish	Ectotherm	Carnivore	Conservation
Fish	Marine: salmon, tuna, shark	Ectotherm	Carnivore	Control
Fish	Fresh water: catfish, trout	Ectotherm	Omnivore	Control
Amphibian	Frogs, salamanders	Ectotherm	Carnivore	Conservation
Reptile	Snakes, lizards, crocodiles	Ectotherm	Carnivore	Conservation
Reptile	Iguanine lizards, chelonians	Ectotherm	Herbivore	Conservation
Bird	Passerines: songbirds	Endotherm	Omnivore	Conservation
Bird	Ratites: emus, ostrich, rhea	Endotherm	Omnivore	Control
Bird	Upland game birds: grouse, ptarmigan, phesants	Endotherm	Herbivore	Control
Bird	Waterfowl: geese, and ducks	Endotherm	Herbivore	Control
Bird	Seabirds: waders, albatross, gulls	Endotherm	Carnivore	Conservation
Bird	Crane, raptors	Endotherm	Carnivore	Conservation
Mammal	Marine: seals, whales	Endotherm	Carnivore	Conservation
Mammal	Marsupials: grazing kangaroos	Endotherm	Herbivore	Control
Mammal	Marsupials: wallabies, wombats, possums	Endotherm	Herbivore	Conservation
Mammal	Marsupials: bandicoots, quolls	Endotherm	Carnivore	Conservation
Mammal	Rodents	Endotherm	Omnivore	Control
Mammal	Hares, rabbits	Endotherm	Herbivore	Control
Mammal	Ruminants: deer, sheep, bison, giraffes	Endotherm	Herbivore	Control
Mammal	Horses, rhinos, elephants	Endotherm	Herbivore	Control
Mammal	Primates, lemurs	Endotherm	Omnivore	Conservation
Mammal	Cats: lions, lynx	Endotherm	Carnivore	Conservation
Mammal	Bears, wolves, hyena	Endotherm	Carnivore	Control

* **Source:** Integrative Wildlife Nutrition by P.S.Barboza, K.L.Parker and I.D.Hume published by Springer-Verlag Berlin Heidelberg in 2009; ** **Control**=monitored and often manipulated to control a population for maximum sustainable harvest or minimal adverse effects of overabundance; conservation=monitored and often manipulated to conserve minimal viable population size

ectotherms are usually very close to those of the water. Ectotherms do not require as much food as warm-blooded animals (endotherms) of the same size, but most cannot deal as well with cold surroundings.

Endotherm: Endotherrns are also called warm-blooded animals, i.e., those that maintain a constant body temperature independent of the environment. The endotherms primarily include the birds and mammals; however, some fish are also endothermic. If heat loss exceeds heat generation, metabolism increases to make up the loss or the animal shivers to raise its body temperature. If heat generation exceeds the heat loss, mechanisms such as panting or perspiring increase heat loss. Endotherms can be active and survive at quite low external temperatures (in contrast to ectotherms). Since they must produce heat continuously, they require high quantities of food.

Captive Breeding

Imbalance in eco-system may occur due to death because of natural hazards like earth quakes, poisoning, diseases and poaching and hunting and due to habitat destruction either natural or man-made. The wild animal species may become extinct in the course of time and it is a fact that many species of wild animals are in the stage of extinction. Hence, captive breeding becomes one of the important objectives in case of zoos. It is often becoming a mandatory to have both male and female wild animals of the particular wild animal species under threat. Conservation efforts are directed to protect the wild animals that belong to various species. Hence, zoos, zoological parks and zoological gardens become the better places for the captive breeding of the selected species of wild animals for which the available infrastructures are being utilized.

Mangrove Zoo

A unique 'mangrove zoo' that will display the ecosystem of the Sunderbans will come up at Jharkhali in West Bengal State. Animals found in the mangrove ecosystem such as the Royal Bengal tiger, spotted deer and wild boar, salt-water crocodiles, fishing cats, riverine turtles and otters (*Batagur baska*, semi-aquatic mammals) would be kept at the zoo.

Migratory Birds

Wetlands are home to several rare and migratory birds. One bird is quoted here as an example. During the winter season 'falcons' migrate from South-eastern Siberia and Northern China and stop at Doyang reservoir (Nagaland) each year on their way to Somalia, Kenya and South Africa. Every year, from October to November, they arrive in the northeast, especially in Nagaland for roosting. These 'Amur falcons' are insectivorous. They spend a few days to fatten up for their transoceanic journey to Africa. Trapping of these birds in thousands is reported and are sold for a pittance.

Amur falcons travel up to 22,000 km a year, known to be longest distance migration of birds. Wildlife Institute of India, Dehardun in partnership with other stakeholders tagged five Amur falcons with satellite transmitters in the Doyang area in November, 2013 (Satellite tag with an antenna and solar panel weighing five grams had been fitted on the back of the bird). These satellite transmitters can track their seasonal movements and satellite tagging will bolster conservation efforts initiated by the Nagaland Forest Department and prevent hunting of the migratory birds. They take the route of Wokha in Nagaland, Assam, Bangladesh, the Bay of Bengal, Andhra Pradesh and Karnataka/Maharashtra before entering the airspace over the Arabian Sea to their final destinations.

Similar wetlands elsewhere also attract the migratory birds in the season. Some of the commonly seen migratory birds are open-bill stork, night heron, grey heron, pond heron or paddy bird, grey pelican, little cormorants, spoonbill, little egret, large egret, cattle egret, white ibis, shoveller duck, dab chick, Indian moorhen and darters or snake bird.

Control and Conservation of Wildlife

As the human population continued to grow, wild animal populations declined (due to shrinking habitats), with some of these now officially designated as threatened or endangered. Such endangered species include the Asiatic lion, Asian elephant, tiger, white-rumped vulture, Asian one-horned rhinoceros and water buffalo. There is a vast array of reptiles, birds and amphibians that are slowly disappearing too. In the best interests of society, more intensive management of wildlife populations and habitat is necessary. Man-animal conflicts are happening frequently in the forest-adjoining areas. Lack of feed and water cause the wild animals to intrude into human habitations. Killing people and causing damage to croplands in those forest-adjoining areas are sometimes common in the present times. Indian gaurs are kept at bay by hanging saris along the fence of farmlands, in one of these areas.

Many birds and animals are killed for their horns (rhino) or tusks (elephants); or for their flesh to gain from the aphrodisiac properties or a cure for asthma etc. Black naped hares are trapped by the poachers. These are the main prey for jungle cats, mongoose, jackels and foxes. If hare population gets dwindled, the survival of small mammals would be affected very badly.

Steps Initiated for Conservation

India has a long history of conservation with national parks and protected areas springing up as early as 1935.The Indian Board for Wildlife is the main advisory board for advising the Government of India regarding the wildlife policy in the country. It was set up in 1952 to prevent the extinction of animal and bird species. In recent years many of the International Bodies like International Union for Conservation of Nature and Natural Resources (IUCN; now called as World Conservation Union), World Wildlife Fund International (WWF) and International Council for Bird Preservation (ICBP) have come up for purposes of safe guarding conservation, management and creation of awareness, and India is a member of all these bodies. For effective conservation of wildlife three basic needs should be fulfilled, *viz* adequate feed and water, place of refuge and place to breed in safely.

At present, India has more than 600 protected areas with the Ministry of Environment and Forest working with the objective of protecting wildlife, controlling poaching, smuggling and illegal trade in wildlife through the landmark Wildlife Protection Act of 1972. Wildlife Institute of India was established in Dehradun in 1982 as a centre for wildlife training, research, publication and extension in India. World wildlife week is celebrated from October 2 to 8. It is an annual event aims to raise awareness about the conservation of wildlife

Schedules of Wildlife Protection Act, 1972

There are six schedules from I to VI. Wildlife Protection Act 1972 has amendments during 1986, 1991and 2002. Hunting of wild animals is prohibited. No person shall hunt any wild animal specified in Schdule I, II, III and IV (as per Section 9 of the Act) except as provided under Section 11 and Section 12 (Chief Wildlife Warden may permit to hunt any wild animal specified in Schdule I as per these Sections).

Schedule I

Rare and endangered species which are totally protected -

Part I - Mammals (from 1 to 41): Andaman wild pig, bharal, binturong, black buck, brow-antlered deer or thanmin, himalayan brown bear, capped langur, caracal, catacean spp, cheetah, chinese pangolin, chinkara or indian gazelle, clouded leopard, crab-eating macaque, desert cat, desert fox, dugong, ermine, fishing cat, four-horned antelope, cagetic dolphin, gaur or Indian bison, golden cat, golden langur, Himalayan ibex, Himalayan tahr, hispid hare, hog badger, hoolock gibbon, Indian elephant, Indian lion, Indian wild ass, Indian wolf, Kashmir stag, leaf monkey, leopard or panther, leopard cat, lesser or red panda, Lion-tailed macaque, Loris, little Indian porpoise, lynx, Malabar civet, malay or sun bear, marbled cat, markhor mouse deer, musk deer, Nilgiri Tahr, Niligiri langur, nayan or great Tibetan sheep, pallas' cat, pangolin, pygmy hog, ratel, Indian one-horned Rhinoceros, Rusty spotted cat, Serow, clawless otter, sloth bear, slow loris, small Travancore flying squirrel, snow leopard, snubfin dolphin, spotted linsang, Swamp deer, takin or mishmi takin, Tibetan fox, Tibetan gazelle, Tibetan wild ass, tiger, urial or shapu, wild buffalo, wild yak and Tibetan wolf.

Part II - Amphibians and Reptiles (from 1 to 14): Audithia turtle, barred, oval, or yellow monitor lizard, crocodiles, terrapin, eastern hill terrapin, gharial, ganges soft-shelled turtle, golden gecko, green sea turtle, hawksbill turtle, indian egg-eating snake, inidian soft-shelled turtle, kerala forest terrapin, leathery turtle, oliverback loggerhead turtle, peacock-marked soft-shelled turtle, Pythons, sail terrapin and spotted black terrapin.

Part II A - Fishes (from 1 to 4): Whale shark, Shark and Ray (nine species), Sea horse and Giant grouper.

Part III - Birds (from 1 to 18): Andaman teal, Assam bamboo partridge, bazas, Bengal florican, black-necked crane, blood pheasants, cheer pheasant, eastern white stork, forest spotted owlet, frogmouths, great Indian bustard, great Indian hornbill, hawks, hooded crane, hornbills, houbara bustard, hume's bar-backed pheasant, Indian pied hornbill, jerdon's courser, lammergeyer, large falcons, large whistling teal, lesser florican, monal pheasants, mountain quail, narcondam hornbill, nicobar megapode, nicobar pigeon, osprey or fish eating eagle, peacock pheasants, peafowl, pink-headed duck, scalater's monal, Siberian white crane, Tibetan snow cock, tragopan pheasants, white-bellied sea eagle, white-eared pheasants, white spoonbill and white-winged wood duck.

Part IV -Crustacea and Insects: Butterflies and Moths.

Part IV A - Coelentrates (from 1 to 5): Roof building coral, Black coral, Organ pipe coral, Fire coral and Sea fan.

Part IV B - Mollusca (from 1 to 9)

Part IV C - Echinodermata: Sea cucumber (all Holothurians)

Schedule II

'Game' species which have been given more stringent protection -

Part I (from 1 to 25) - assamese macaque, Bengal porcupine, Bonnet macaque, Cetatean spp. Common langur, ferret badgers, Himalayan crestless porcupine, Himalayan newt or salamander, pig-tailed macaque, rhesus macaque, stump-tailed macaque, Wild dog or dhole, Chameleon and Spiny-tailed lizard or Sanda.

Part II (from 1 to 15) - Beetles; civets (all species of Viverridae except Malabar civet), common fox, flying squirrels, giant squirrels, Himalayan black bear, jackal , jungle cat, marmots, martens, otters, pole cats, red fox, sperm whale, easels, checkered keelback snake, dhaman or rat snake, dog-faced water snake, Indian cobras, king cobra, oliveceous keelback snake, russel's viper and varanus species (excluding yellow monitor lizard).

Schedule III

'Game' species: These are Barking deer or Muntjac, chital or spotted deer, Gorals, Hog deer, hyaena, Nilgai, sambar, wild pig and Sponges.

Schedule IV: 'Game' species

Five-striped palm squirrel, hares (Black naped hare, Common Indian hare, Desert hare, Himalayan mouse hare), Hedgehogs, Indian porcupine, Mongooses (All species of genus Herpestes)

Birds other than those, which appear in other schedules (1 to 80)

Snakes other than those species listed in Schedule I, part II; and Schedule II, part II

Fresh water frogs, three-keeled turtle, tortoises, viviparous toads, voles and certains families of butterflies and moths and Mollusca

Schedule V: Vermin

Common crow, Fruit bats, Mice and Rats

Schedule VI

Beddomes' cycad, Kuth, Picher plant, Ladies slipper orchids, Red Vanda, Blue Vanda

"Captive animal" means any animal, specified in Schedule I, Schedule II, Schedule III or Schedule IV, which is captured or kept or bred in captivity.

Immunization of livestock: (1) The Chief Wildlife Warden shall take such measures in such manner as may be prescribed, for immunization against communicable diseases of the livestock kept in or within five kilometers of the sanctuary. (2) No person shall take, or cause to be taken or graze, any livestock in a sanctuary without getting it immunized (Section 33A).

Common Wild Animals in Indian Zoos

Commonly held carnivores: Lion, tiger, panther, jungle cat, hyena, jackals, wild dog, otter, fox, wolf, jaguar etc.

Other wild animals: Gaur, wild pig, nilgai, spotted deer, sambar deer, porcupine, sloth bear, giant squirrels, zebra, Indian pangolin, hog badger, kangaroo, rhinoceros, giraffe etc.

Reptiles: Cobra, king cobra, russels wiper, rat snake, green snake, krait, reticulated python, rock python, monitor lizard, Indian soft shelled turtle, mugger, gharial etc.

Aviary species: Peacocks, cockatoo, cockatiel, African grey parrot, grey horn bills, rosy pelicans, painted storks, budgerigars, love birds, swan, egrets, born owls, vultures, kites, shikara etc.

Endangered Wild Animal Species in India

Endangered wild animals are those whose numbers are at a critically low level and whose habitats are so drastically reduced or damaged that they are in imminent danger of extinction. The International Union for Conservation of Nature and Natural Resources (IUCN) maintains a Red Data Book providing a record of animals that are known to be in danger. Schedule I of Indian Wildlife Protection Act 1972 list out the rare and endangered wild animal species that are governed by significant legal status.

Ex-situ Conservation Programme

The Anna Arignar Zoological Park, popularly known as Vandalur zoo, is spread across 602 hectares and is home to 1,541 animals. Now it is proposed to set up 'the Advanced Institute of Wildlife Conservation Centre (AIWCC)' to conduct research on rare species, especially endangered ones specifically on 13 indigenous species. These include lion-tailed macaque (LTM), nilgiri langur, elephants, tigers and black sheep.

Ex-situ conservation programme is being implemented to revive and regenerate certain wildlife species that are under conservation programme. For example, in case of Asian rhino, the programme aims to have at least 100 healthy rhinos be bred in captivity. Assam State Zoo, Delhi Zoo and Patna Zoo are involved in rhino ex-situ conservation. Assam zoo has also been selected for ex-situ conservation programme of serow, golden langur, golden cat and grey peacock pheasant.

Food Chain - Energy and Nutrient Flow Through Ecosystem

Food chains are the routes taken by energy and nutrients through an ecosystem. The link begins with producers (green plants), then advance to primary consumers (herbivores), and go on to secondary consumers (predators). Grasses are the producer trophic in a prairie ecosystem, and bison represents the primary consumers. Wolves preying on bison become secondary consumers in this food chain.

Less energy is available at each successive trophic level in an ecosystem. Thus, when measured per unit of area, there is more energy in green plants than in herbivores and more in herbivores than in primary carnivores and so on. Hence, wildlife managers cannot expect larger number of mink (*Mustela vision*), which are predators, than of muskrats, which are herbivores, irrespective of the demands of trappers and the market place.

Human manipulations alter the patterns in which energy and matter flow through ecosystem. Effective wildlife nutritional management involves recognition of the degree to which communities are disrupted when plant and animal populations are manipulated. These activities should not unduly disrupt the overall functioning of communities in which wildlife management is practiced.

Here an example is depicted how the very survival of tiger is threatened. Lantana is a major invasive plant that spreads over the native grass species in certain forests and creates a mat like structure. This will not allow the plants to regenerate. Thus lantana plant smothers the native species of grasses, plants and shrubs. The moisture in the ground is sucked by lantana, making the place dry. During the dry season a small fire in the dry patch of lantana will result in a forest fire, destroying vegetation, birds, animals and smaller life forms. Spreading of lantana will destroy and degrade the biodiversity. In this process, herbivores such as Indian gaur, spotted deer, sambar will not get the required grass, shrubs or other plants for their feeding. If herbivores are affected, the predators such as tiger and leopard will die of starvation. It poses a severe threat to the very survival of tiger, the apex species in the food chain. Hence the predators enter human habitations for food.

Lizards are ectotherms (meaning their activity depends on their external temperature) and their survival is threatened because of global warming. The disappearance of the lizard population is likely to cause a break in the food chain. Lizards are important prey for many birds, snakes and other animals, while lizards predate on insects.

Productivity Gradient of Wildlife

Nutrition is the process whereby the animal procures feeds from its external environment and processes them for the continued functioning of internal metabolism. All animals are located somewhere on a tissue metabolism gradient (Figure 1). The position of an animal along the gradient represents a dynamic balancing between cellular and organismal requirements and the rate and efficiency at which specific components of the external environment can be acquired.

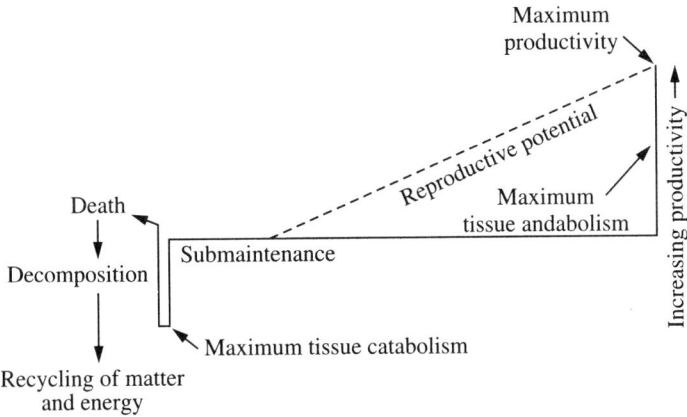

Figure 1   The productivity gradient experienced by all wildlife (Moen, 1973)

Animal tissues decompose and return their nutrients to soils and the plants grow on these nutrients. Soils-Plants-Animals exist as the cycle of nutrition continues. Our ability to effectively conserve and manage wildlife species depends on understanding their needs in changing habitats with changing food supplies.

Wildlife Diversity and Population Density - Environmental Influence

Wildlife diversity and abundance are high in rainforest ecosystems that are characterized by moderate temperature and high availability of water and nutrients that promote continuous plant production. Conversely, hot deserts typically support smaller populations of fewer species of wildlife because temperature and precipitation are highly variable and less conducive to plant production.

There are concerns about animal populations. Animals depend on nutrient resources in their habitat. Animals have to contend with variations in the supply of resources and the environmental challenges in their habitat. Resource supply and demand are features of both the environment and wildlife. The environment supplies feed but also exert demands on the animal. For example, low ambient temperatures increase the demand for energy to heat the body whereas high ambient temperatures increase the need for water to cool the animal. The demands of the animal for maintenance, growth and reproduction are ultimately met with feed from the environment.

8

Taxonomy of Wild Animals and Birds

Taxonomy of Wild Mammals

The taxonomy in wild mammals consists of many orders and families. The binomial nomenclature of the Swedish naturalist Carolus Linnaeus is followed in the animal kingdom. Genus name is followed by species name in general.

Mammalians are divided into three classes: (I) Allotheria (extinct), (II) prototheria (includes primitive mammals) and (III) theria (includes most of the mammals).

(II) Prototheria: Order Monotremata - these animals have the following features. Testes are abdominal and cloaca is present. Mammary glands are present without nipples. They lack external ear. Examples: Spiny anteater/Echidna and Duck billed platypus

(III) Theria has three subclasses: (A) Pantotheria (extinct), (B) metatheria and (C) eutheria.

(B) Metatheria: This group consists of a single order Marsupilia. Marsupials are the animals with a brood pouch or marsupium on the abdomen of the females in which the new born is taken care of well. Examples: Kangaroo, tiger cat, opossum and the like. Young ones are born prematurely after a short gestation. Hence they are nurtured in the marsupium. Mammary gland opens by nipples into the marsupium. They are strictly herbivores and are very fond of grasses with very few carnivore species. They are pre-gastric fermenters.

(C) Eutheria: Young ones born in advanced stage after a long gestation. These animals lack marsupium and cloaca. This group comprises all other mammals that are again divided into many orders: Edentata, Pholidota, Primates, Proboscidea, Lagomorpha, Dermoptera, Chiroptera, Insectivora,

Rodentia, Hyracoidea, Tubelidentata, Artiodactyla, Perissodactyla, Carnivora, Cetacea, Pinnipedia and Sirenia.

1. **Order proboscidea:** Presence of large muscular proboscis is the characteristic of this order. Proboscis has nose and upper lip. Two upper incisors are elongated as tusks. Canines are absent. Two species of elephants are in existence: African elephant (Loxodonta africana) -There are two sub-species in the African elephants: Smaller forest elephant and the larger bush or savannah elephant; Asiatic elephant (Eliphas maximus)-There are four sub-species in the Asiatic elephants: Indian, Ceylon, Sumatran and Malaysian.

2. **Order logomorpha:** The lagomorphs have long hind limbs used for jumping. Family Leporidae consists of rabbit and hare. Family Ochotonide consists of mouse-hare. Coprophagy and caecotrophy are common practice.

3. **Order dermoptera:** Example - flying or gliding lemur or Colugo

4. **Order chiroptera:** Example - bats- some are frugivorous while some eat insects and forage at night.

5. **Order insectivora:** Very primitive small mammals, covered with spines or fur. Eight families: Solenodons, Tenrecs, African water shrews, Golden moles, Hedgehogs, Elephant shrews, True shrews, True moles. In the insectivores, the hedgehogs and tenrecs have more spines on skin and the spiny nature helps them to roll like balls when the predators attempt to attack them. Such anatomical variants vary from species to species.

6. **Rodentia order** is the largest order of mammals. It is divided into three suborders. (1) Sciuromorpha ("Squirrellike") examples include squirrels, marmots, chipmunks, gophers, beavers, kangaroo rats, springhaas. (2) Myomorpha ("ratlike") examples include rat, mice, voles, hamsters, lemmings. (3) Hystricomorpha ("porcupinelike") examples include porcupines, cavies, capybaras, chinchillas, agoutis. Other species belong to rodentia order are Tuco-tucos, Nutria, Guinea pig, woodchuck, Pacas, Pacarana, Eastern fox squirrel, burrowing rodents like woodchuck or groundhog etc.

7. **Order artiodactylids:** This order consists of two sub orders.

(1) **Bunodontia:** Includes pigs and allies; suidae (old world pigs), tayassuidae (new world pigs), hippopotamidae (horse of the river; feed on aquatic plants)

(2) **Pseudoruminants:** Family Tragulidae-e.g., mouse deer; family Camelidae: pseudoruminant because omasum is rudimentary and the presence of incisors; have soft and broad feet with no hoof; e.g., llama and alpaca.

(3) **Pecora:** Ruminants

(i) **Giraffidae:** Examples giraffe and okapi: Both species have the elongated neck but the neck of the giraffe is longer than that of okapi.

(ii) **Antelopes and gazelles:** The antelopes and gazelles are called as the earliest ruminants. Blackbuck (Antelope cervipara): The horns are spiral in nature. The Indian races are attractive to look at. Four horned antelope (Tetracerus quadricornis) are also called as Chowsingha. Chinkara or Indian gazelle: The Horns of the males are ringed, while the females are smooth and at times, the females are hornless too.

(iii) **Cervids:** Antlers are the anatomical specialty of these animals. Various species of deer are farmed in many countries. The antlers are harvested in a systematic manner for medicinal purposes. Spotted deer or chital: These are the most sociable animal of all the deer. Sambar deer, swamp deer or barasingha, hog deer, musk deer (There is no antler in these animals; musk gland is located below the abdomen skin in male), mouse deer or Indian chevrotain (smallest deer in India) are other examples.

(iv) **Bovids:** This is the largest group of artiodactyla and has variety of animals. Wild oxen: The significant are Gaur or Indian bison, wild buffalo, yak. Nilgai: The male animals are called as blue bulls. Wild goat: Nilgiri tahr

8. **Order perissodactylids:** Families equidae (equids), tapiridae (tapirs) and rhinocerotidae (rhinoceroses)

9. **Order carnivora:** Fissipedia is the sub-order that comprises most known terrestrial carnivorous wild animals like lion, tiger, panther, wolf, hyaena, wild dog, jackals etc.

Jackals (*Canis aureus*): Jackals are present throughout India in small number on any kind of habitat ranging from humid dense forests to dry open plains. This animal comes out during the dusk and retires by dawn. This can make a typical howl that is long drawn and high pitched one. Dead carcasses are eaten by them and jackals also feed on weak livestock and poultry.

Indian foxes (*Vulpes bengalensis*): Foxes are the small slim animals with slender limbs. These are seen in agricultural fields and are solitary hunters but appear to tolerate the presence of common mongoose near its den.

Wolf (*Canis lupus*): Wolf is seen in several parts of India. These animals assume a height of about 65-75 cm and the weight of these carnivores may be about 18-28Kg.

Hyaenas: Hyaenas have large anal glands and are scavengers. They are nocturnal in nature and are stocky dog like animals inhabiting the plains of southwest Asia and Africa. They walk on toes, four on each foot.

The families in Carnivora order are (1). Canidae - wild dogs, jackal, fox, wolf (2). Felidae - Tiger, lion, panther, jungle cat, caracal and jaguars, leaopard cat (3). Ursidae - Bears (4). Mustelidae - Skinks, Otters, weasels (5). Viverridae - Mongooses, Civets (6). Procyonidae - Raccoons, Kinkajou, pandas (7). Hyaenidae - Hyaenas - striped hyaena is the only species available in India.

Other felids have also to be understood in terms of conservation of wild fauna: Clouded leopard (*Neofelis nebulosa*): These animals are seen in Assam and Sikkim. Cheetah or Hunting leopard (*Acinonyx jubatus*): Cheetah is extinct in India, at present. Caracal and Jaguars: Caracals are seen in north and north-west hills of Cutch and Jaguars are considered to be the sturdy animals. Lynx (*Felis lynx*): Lynx are seen in upper Indus valley, Ladak, Gilgit and Tibet. These animals are called as "isabellina". Indian desert cat: Indian desert cats are seen in deserts of north -western India extending to the drier regions of Central India. Marbled cat (*Felis marmorata*): Marbled cats are sighted in Sikkim and Assam. Single race occurs in India. Leopard cat (*Felis bengalensis*): Leopard cats can be sighted in wider parts of India from Kashmir to Cape Camorin. Golden cat (*Felis temmincki*): In Assam and Sikkim, Golden cats are present. Pallas cat (*Felis manul*): Pallas cats are seen in Ladak

Viverrids: Most of the viverrids have scent glands in the anal region that can emit a strong smelling fluid and it is called as 'civet'. These materials are having pheromone like effects. Some of the species such as Common palm civet (Toddy cat), small Indian civet, common mongoose are distributed throughout India.

Ursids: The bears have a compact body with a short neck and quadrupedal gait. However, they are capable of standing like human and are prone for stereotypical behaviour if left uncared or bored. These animals are exploited in circuse events etc. Bears are exceedingly dangerous in nature. Bears are usually solitary in nature.

Important species of bears: Sloth bear (Melursus ursinus), Asiatic bear (Selenarctos thibetanus), Spectacled bear (Tremarctos arnatus), Malayan sun bear (Helarctos malayanus), Polar bear (Thalarctos maritimus), Alaskan brown bear (Ursus arctos), American black bear (Ursus americanus)

Marine Mammals

10. **Order cetacea:** Commonly live in sea but few live in fresh water also. They are carnivorous and predaceous. Includes whales (100 feet), dolphins (five feet) and porpoises.

11. **Order Pinnipedia:** Examples include seals, walruses and sea-lions (marine carnivores). They are slow and clumsy on land where they come to rest and raise their young ones.

12. **Order Sirenia:** Durong or sea cows and manatees

Marine mammals that spend large time in marine environment: Polar bears (carnivores falling in Ursidae family) and sea otters (carnivores belonging to family Ursidae)

Taxonomy of Reptiles

Birds and mammals have evolved from reptiles. Reptiles are the ectothermic animals and air breathing vertebrates. Turtles are the most ancient reptiles and the snakes the most recent. Since the reptiles share many anatomical features with bird, both the reptile and birds are sometimes considered together in the single group entitled as "Sauropsida". It consists of chelonians, crocodiles, lizards, snakes etc. Reptiles are seen in all continents except Antarctica and on most islands.

Majority of the reptiles are carnivorous especially the snakes (Marine Green turtle and Green Iguana are herbivores). They either lay egg or give birth to young but in both instances the embryo, like that of a mammal is enclosed in an amnion. Whether hatched from an egg or born alive, the reptiles don't pass through a larval stage or undergo metamorphosis as do amphibians. Reptiles are capable of growth throughout the life. Dry water-proof skins with horny scales are present. Scales are not separated as seen in fish but they are folds of skin.

Orders and sub-orders in Reptiles: There are three orders in reptilian group: (1) Testudinata (Chelonia) - This group comprises turtles, tortoises, terrapins and sea-turtles; (2) Crocodilia - This group comprises crocodiles, caimans, alligators and gavials; (3) Squamata - This group comprises lizards and snakes. Sub-orders: Amphisbaenia (e.g., Worm lizards), Sphenodontia (e.g., Tuatara in Newzealand), Serpentes (Ophidia) (e.g., Snakes) and Lacertilia (Sauria) (e.g., Lizards)

Alligators and Crocodiles

All alligators are crocodiles, but not all crocodiles are alligators. Both belong to the reptilian order Crocodylia. But alligators belong to Alligatoridae family and crocodiles to Crocodylidae family.

Alligators have broad-heads and rounded snouts, while crocodiles have triangular-shaped heads and pointed snouts. When mouth is closed, both the enlarged teeth on each side of the crocodile's lower jaw are plainly visible, while they fit into pits in the upper jaw (and are not visible) in the alligator.

Crocodilians (alligator, crocodile and gharial or gavial) are ideally suited for life in water and on land. They are most at home in the water and can hold their breath for up to an hour. Eyes situated atop their heads enable them to keep a lookout for prey, while their powerful tails swiftly propel them through the water. They also have night vision. Their ears are sensitive enough to hear offspring calling from inside their eggs. Sense of smell is also highly developed due to special organs in their snouts.

Crocodiles and alligators are top-notch hunters and will eat just about anything they can get their teeth on, from fish and turtle to monkeys and buffalo. With teeth specialized for spearing, they can swallow large chunks or the entire animal whole without chewing it.

Taxonomy of Birds

Kingdom:	Animalia
Phylum:	Chordata
Class:	Aves
Order:	
Family:	
Genus:	
Species:	

Some common birds

Sl No	Common name	Zoological name	Classification Order	Family
1	House crow Corvus splendens	*Passeriformes*	Corvidae	
2	Jungle crow	*Corvus macrorhynchos*	Passeriformes	Corvidae
3	Indian treepie	*Dendrocitta vagabunda*	Passeriformes	Corvidae
4	Indian pitta	*Pitta brachyura*	Passeriformes	Pittidae

5	Black drongo	*Dicrurus macrocercus*	Passeriformes	Dicrurudae
6	Common myna	*Acridotheres tristis*	Passeriformes	Sturnidae
7	Spotted munia	*Lonchra punctulata*	Passeriformes	Estreldidae
8	Black-headed munia	*L.malacca*	Passeriformes	Estreldidae
9	Zebra Finch	*Taeniopygia guttata*	Passeriformes	Estrildidae
10	Bengalese Finch	*Lonchura striata*	Passeriformes	Estrildidae
11	House sparrow	*Passer domesticus*	Passeriformes	Passeridae
12	Small minivet	*Pericrocotus cinnamomeus*	Passeriformes	Camphiphagiidae
13	Asian paradise -flycatcher	*Terpsiphone paradise*	Passeriformes	Monarchidae
14	Grey francolin	*Francolinus pondicerianus*	Galliformes	Phasianidae
15	Indian peafowl	*Pavo cristatus*	Galliformes	Phasianidae
16	Common hoopoe	*Upupa epops*	Upupiformes	Upupidae
17	Small blue kingfisher	*Alcedo atthis*	Coraciiformes	Alcedinidae
18	Pied crested cuckoo	*Clamater jacobinus*	Cuculiformes	Cuculidae
19	Drongo cuckoo	*Surniculus lugubris*	Cuculiformes	Centropodidae
20	Asian palm swift	*Cypsiurus balasiensis*	Apodiformes	Apodidae
21	Eastern grass owl	*Tyto longimembris*	Strigiformes	Tytonidae
22	Blue rock pigeon	*Columbia livia*	Columbiformes	Columbidae
23	Spotted dove	*Streptopelia chinensis*	Columbiformes	Columbidae
24	Shikra	*Accipiter badius*	Falconiformes	Accipitridae

Some common birds from Psittaciformes Order

Sl No	Common name	Zoological name	Order	Family
1	Chattering Lory	Lorius garrulus	Psittaciformes	Psittacidae
2	Eclectus parrot	Eclectus roratus	Psittaciformes	Psittacidae
3	Green winged Macaw	Ara chloroptera	Psittaciformes	Psittacidae
4	Sulphur Crested Cockatoo	Cacatua sulphurea	Psittaciformes	Psittacidae
5	Great White cockatoo	Cacatua alba	Psittaciformes	Psittacidae
6	African Grey Parrot	Psittacus erithacus	Psittaciformes	Psittacidae
7	Rainbow Lory	Trichoglossus haemadotus	Psittaciformes	Psittacidae
8	Alexandrine Parakeet	Psittacula eupatria	Psittaciformes	Psittacidae
9	Plum headed Parakeet	Psittacula cyanocephala	Psittaciformes	Psittacidae
10	Rose-ringed parakeet	Psittacula krameri	Psittaciformes	Psittacidae
11	Grey Cockatiel	Nymphicus hollandicus	Psittaciformes	Psittacidae

12	Pied Cockatiel	*Nymphicus hollandicus*	Psittaciformes	Psittacidae
13	Lutino Cockatiel	*Nymphicus hollandicus*	Psittaciformes	Psittacidae
14	Masked Love bird	*Agapornis personata personata*	Psittaciformes	Psittacidae
15	Fischer's Lovebird	*Agapornis personata fischeri*	Psittaciformes	Psittacidae
16	Peach faced Love bird	*Agapornis roseicollis*	Psittaciformes	Psittacidae
17	Lutino budgerigar	*Melopsittacus undulatus*	Psittaciformes	Psittacidae
18	Albino budgerigar	*Melopsittacus undulatus*	Psittaciformes	Psittacidae
19	Scarlet Macaw	*Ara macao*	Psittaciformes	Psittacidae
20	Sun Conure	*Aratinga solstitialis*	Psittaciformes	Psittacidae

9

Nutritional Classification of Animals

Animal species can be grouped into classes based on the main types of food they voluntarily eat. There are three major classes: carnivores, omnivores and herbivores.

Carnivores

Carnivores are meat-eaters (faunivores or animal-eaters), insect-eaters (insectivores) and fish-eaters (piscivores). The spotted-tailquoll (*Dasyurus maculate*) eats only meat and has been called a 'hypercarnivore' or specialist carnivore.

Omnivores

Omnivores have a dietary range that includes foods of both vegetable and animal origins.

Herbivores

Herbivores eat plants and include animals which eat predominantly seeds (granivores), fruit (frugivores) and plant leaves (folivores or graminivores). The Koala (*Phascolarctos cinereus*) is a specialist herbivore and eats only the leaves of a few eucalyptus species. Herbivores need plants for food, and in response plants have defenses against animal predators. But they also exploit animals and in turn are dependent on animals for such things as seed dispersal and recycling of nutrients.

Herbivores evolved several nutritional strategies to exploit the plant food resources. 1. These include extraction of energy in cellulosic matter [dominated by grazing ruminants] and selective feeding for highly and rapidly digestible plant parts [dominated by small ruminants]. 2. Many of these small ruminants have developed salivary or ruminal metabolic adaptations [e.g., tannin-binding salivary mucins] to cope with tannins and other secondary substances. 3. Consuming large quantity of feed with low energy extraction. This is exclusively a domain of certain non-ruminants. The largest herbivores are non-ruminants. It appears the specialization of grazing ruminants allows a smaller animal to achieve the digestive capacity of larger non-ruminants (Van Soest et al., 1995).

Classification of Herbivores

There is considerable variation in the ways in which herbivores are classified. 1. Non-ruminant herbivore 2. Ruminant herbivore

Morphophysiological feeding types among the herbivores: Hoffman classified the herbivorous mammals into **three classes** (concentrate selectors, grass and roughage eaters and mixed feeders) based on their feeding preferences (R.R.Hofman, 1988) while P.J.Van Soest's view of classification of herbivores is furnished in Table 2.

Table 2. Classification of herbivores (Source: P.J.Van Soest (1994) p.27)

Class	Ruminants	Non-ruminants
Concentrate selector		
Fruit and foliage selectors	Duikers, sunis, gerenuk	Rabbits Sumatran, black rhinoceros
Tree and shrub browsers	Deer, giraffe, kudus	—
Intermediate feeders		
Prefer forbs or browsing	Moose, goats, elands, gazelles	—
Prefer grass	Sheep, impalas	—
Bulk and roughage eaters		
Fresh grass grazers	Buffaloes, cattle, gnus, kobs, oribis	Hippopotamus
Roughage grazers	Hartebeests, topis	Horses, elephants, white and Indian rhinos, zebras
Dry region grazers	Oryxes, camels, roan and sable antelope	Kangaroos

Non-ruminant Herbivores

Pregastric fermenters: Examples are kangaroos, wallabies, peccaries, hippopotamuses and certain primates (langur, colobus and proboscis monkeys). They have a voluminous compartmentalized or sacculated forestomach. The forestomach fermentation chamber is approximately 86, 92 and 95% total weight of gastrointestinal tract in peccaries, kangaroos and hippopotamus, respectively. The process of regurgitation and remastication is known as merycism in non-ruminants.

Hindgut fermenters: Examples are horse, ass, zebra, elephant, rabbit, hare, rhinoceros and certain primates (howler monkeys, marmosets, galagos). They have capacious, sacculated large intestine and compartmentalized caecum. These animals may be called as caecal fermenters. Wild pigs have moderately large caecum, but a very large sacculated colon (colon fermenters). Significant amount of microbial fermentation takes place in the hind gut. Post gastric fermenters depend on large intestine for digestion of fibre.

These herbivores increase consumption to overcome the limitation of low digestibility. They sacrifice retention time to utilize cell contents. Elephant is the largest living herbivore. The elephant has fast passage and lives on bulk, i.e. roughage, and low extraction of energy i.e. low digestibility. The herbivorous dinosaurs (50-ton body weight) might have the same strategy. The hindgut content in caecum and colon of an elephant is 11% (Van Hoven et al., 1981). Energy derived from the large intestine can meet 100, 26-30 and 30% of dietary energy requirement in elephant, monkey and wild hare (Van Hoven et al., 1981, Milton, 1981), respectively (see also Table 2 in chapter 10, page no. 139).

Ruminant Herbivores

The range in mature size of living ruminants is from about 3-1000 kg, and constitutes a range of feeding behaviours. Small body size [relative to food] will allow an animal to pick and select. Large size has implications for increased digestive capacity. Large ruminants retain the fibrous grasses more time in the gastrointestinal tract and hence they have restricted forage intake. They have the potential capacity for greater retention and extraction of energy.

Below 30 kg of body size there is an increasing pressure for selective feeding. High digestibility and retention times in five species [asian mouse deer, 2.8kg; pudu, 9.1kg; maxwell's duiker, 9.4kg; bay duiker, 12.1kg;

brocket, 20.2kg] of very small ruminants are reported (Van Soest et al., 1995). These small animals are believed to be largely frugivorous with varying consumption of browse or foliage in their native habitats. These animals selectively consumed the ones with lower lignification and higher rates of digestion. Thus they could grow and reproduce in their natural habitat. It is reported that only pectins and unlignified primary cell walls of vegetables can have rates of digestion greater than 15%/h needed by growing and lactating animals in the 10 kg size range.

Herbivores: Foregut and hindgut fermenters

Herbivores may also be classified based on the site of fermentation in the gastrointestinal tract. Herbivores are either foregut or hindgut fermenters

The foregut fermenters include the macropods (e.g. kangaroos, wallabies), the camelids (e.g. camels, llamas, alpacas), some suids (hippopotamus) and the ruminants (e.g. sheep, goats, cattle, buffaloes, deer). All these animals have a large organ anterior to the gastric stomach where microbial fermentation occurs. This allows them to benefit from the microbial digestion of forage cell walls before feed passes into the true stomach and intestines for further digestion.

The hindgut fermenters have a greatly enlarged caecum, or a greatly enlarged colon, or both. They subject their feed to gastric and small intestinal digestion before microbes attack the plant cell wall and any remaining cell contents. Hindgut fermenters are less able to fully digest fibre (plant cell walls) and less able to utilize the B vitamins and amino acids which result from microbial fermentation of feed. Hindgut fermenters have faster rates of passage of feed than ruminants. This can reduce the extent of feed digestion. However, hindgut digestion system can allow these animals to eat larger amounts of less-digestible forages than ruminants. Both horse and koala are able to selectively retain small particles and liquids while voiding larger, possibly indigestible plant fragments. Relative capacity of large intestine is 11-12.5% in ruminant herbivores, 60-65% in non ruminant herbivores, 35-38% in omnivores and 14-16% in carnivores.

Ruminant and Pseudoruminant Animals

Ruminants 'ruminate', i.e. they re-chew undigested forage so that they can increase the rate and extent of digestion in the rumen and promote the escape of undigested and possibly indigestible food pieces from the reticulorumen. Thus, ruminants are cud-chewing, even-toed, hooved animals. Pseudoruminants are cud-chewing animals which have stomachs with three compartments and other minor differences from true ruminants. Taxonomic classification of ruminants and pseudoruminants (Honacki et al., 1982) is presented in Table 3.

Table 3. Taxonomic classification of true ruminants and pseudoruminants

Pseudoruminants

Family - **Tragulidae:** Examples of animals - Mouse deer or Chevrotains. These are small primitive species similar to the pecora (true ruminants) in not having upper incisor teeth and in chewing their cud, but different in that the stomach has only three compartments; males have tusk-like canine teeth.

Family- **Camelidae:** Examples of animals are Camels and camelids (Llamas and related species, Alpaca [Vicugna pacos; Lama pacos]). These animals walk on broad fleshy pads and have two toes on each foot. Their stomachs have only three compartments but have two upper incisor teeth whereas true ruminants have none. Vicugna are unique in the Artiodactyla in that they have ever-growing lower incisors with enamel on only one side. None of these species have horns and they all run with a pacing gait - i.e., by moving the front and rear legs on one side forward in unison.

True ruminants (Pecora)

Suborder: Ruminantia (even-toed, hooved true ruminants)

Family- **Cervidae:** Examples of animals are deer and allied species. These carry antlers (sometimes on both sexes) that comprised of solid bone, which are shed and renewed annually. The musk deer is an exception because it has no antlers; it has enlarged canine teeth which form tusks. The muntjacs have tusks and antlers and tufted deer have tusks and small antlers.

Family- **Giraffidae:** Examples of animals are giraffes and okapi. These are characterized by having short horns covered with hair-bearing skin.

Family- **Bovidae** (ruminants with horn which are shed). Examples of animals are domesticated ruminants, blackbuck or Indian Antelope, bison, mithun, yak, guar.

10

Gastrointestinal Tract of Wild Animals and Birds and Functions

Knowledge of the morphology and functioning of the gastrointestinal tract is essential for understanding nutrient utilization. Digestive systems provide many diverse examples of adaptive ability and function according to the diets. All birds and mammals are dependent on the hydrolysis of ingested organic molecules by gastrointestinal digestive enzymes and the subsequent absorption of small fragments. Fermentative digestion also assumes importance.

Birds

Dietary patterns

The dietary preferences, gastrointestinal tract morphology, and metabolic capabilities of birds have been intimately intertwined during their evolution. The nutrient composition of foods consumed by birds is extremely variable. Trophic-level classification of birds is a useful way to identify morphological convergence due to similar nutritional and ecological parameters.

In general, faunivores (zoophages) consume a diet that is rich in easily digestible protein and fat (animal matter) (see Table 2 and page No 252). Florivores (phytophages) consume diets that are lower in protein and high in carbohydrate (plant matter). At the extremes are piscivores and nectarivores. Fish are composed of mostly protein and fat with less than 1% carbohydrate, whereas nectar is 95% carbohydrate and less than 5% protein and fat. Essentially all important anatomical, physiological, and metabolic systems of the bird's body are adapted to accommodate specialization on these vastly different diets.

Avian Digestive system

The anatomical design of the digestive tract of birds is extremely variable. The line drawings of gastrointestinal tracts of budgerigar, chicken, emu, hawk, hoatzin, and ostrich are presented in the following page for better appreciation. Species consuming easily digested foods (nectar, fruits) have short, simple digestive tracts. Species consuming foods that require more enzymatic attack (animal matter and seeds) have large stomachs and relatively small lower intestines. Some species have digestive tracts dominated by large caeca for the fermentation of plant cell walls, which are difficult to digest.

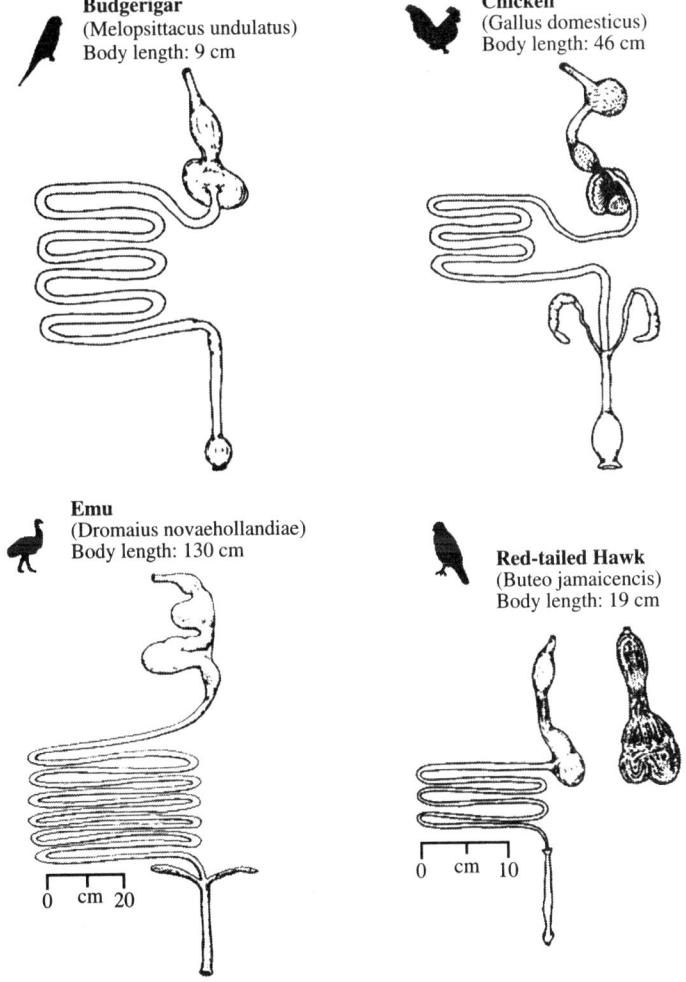

Budgerigar
(Melopsittacus undulatus)
Body length: 9 cm

Chicken
(Gallus domesticus)
Body length: 46 cm

Emu
(Dromaius novaehollandiae)
Body length: 130 cm

0   cm   20

Red-tailed Hawk
(Buteo jamaicencis)
Body length: 19 cm

0   cm   10

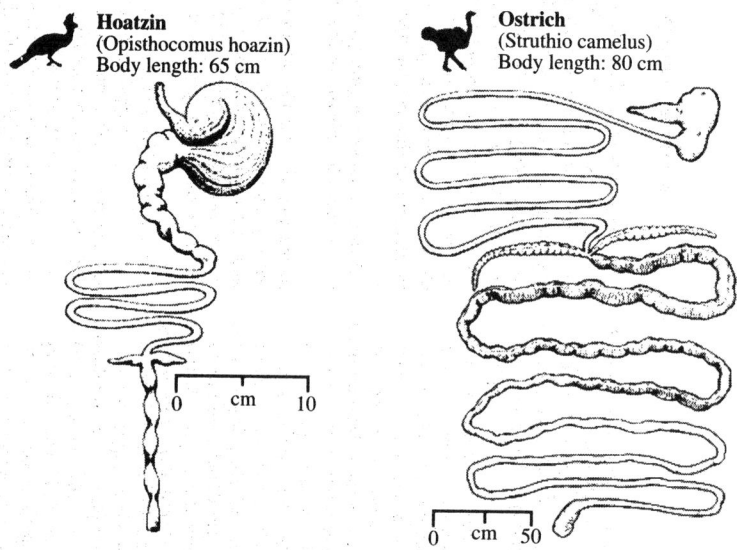

Hoatzin
(Opisthocomus hoazin)
Body length: 65 cm

Ostrich
(Struthio camelus)
Body length: 80 cm

The avian gastrointestinal tract has a greater number of organs than their mammalian counterparts. The avian digestive tract starts with the beak, followed by a toothless mouth, tongue, pharynx, esophagus, crop, proventriculus, ventriculus or gizzard, small intestine, caeca, rectum, cloaca and vent. Accessory organs include the salivary glands, biliary system, pancreas, Peyer's patches, and bursa. The digestive tract is lined with a continuous mucous membrane from the mouth to the vent. This provides protection from abrasion by the food as it passes through and prevents the entry of microorganisms. The intestines are attached to a mesenteric membrane, which contains the blood vessels that perfuse the region of the digestive tract.

Beak

The avian jaw lacks teeth and lips. Birds swallow their food in gulps without chewing. The grasping and particle-size-reduction functions of these structures are taken on by the avian beak, tongue, and gizzard. Earlier, 'beak' was reserved for describing the sharply curved beaks of birds of prey and 'bill' described the broad flat bills of ducks and geese. But the terms 'beak' and 'bill' are often used synonymously in the modern literature. Birds depend on their beaks for acquiring food, but also for preening their feathers, climbing, building nests, defense, and courtship displays. The beak is highly adapted in shape and size according to the type of food that is consumed and how it is processed. It is used to crack and hull seeds, grasp, skim, spear, tear, probe, sieve, etc. The beak is also the entry point of the respiratory system and the upper beak is perforated by the nostrils or nares.

Some examples of specialized beak shapes are mentioned in the following.

- Hornbills and toucans have very large beak; but it is quite light because of vast air-filled cavities strutted with trabeculae.
- White-throated sparrow has light beak adapted for small seeds and plant material.
- Evening grosbeak has heavy beak for cracking seeds with tough coats.
- Atlantic puffin has tall but thin beak for catching and holding small fish.
- Golden-winged warbler has thin beak for gleaning small insects.
- Whimbrel has long beak for probing mud flats for invertebrates.
- Pileated wood pecker has heavy chiseling beak for splintering wood to expose insects.
- Keel-billed toucan has long beak for grasping fruits.
- Great blue heron has long sharp beak for stabbing and spearing small vertebrates.
- Greater flamingo has sharply downturned beak modified into a water filtration system for obtaining small vertebrates.
- Sword-billed hummingbird has extremely long beak for probing deep into tubular-shaped flowers.
- Red-tailed hawk has beak adapted to tearing flesh from small mammals.

Oral Cavity and Pharynx

The oral cavity, or mouth, is between the upper and lower mandibles. The functions of the oral cavity include grasping, testing, mechanical processing, such as crushing or shelling, lubricating, and propelling food into the esophagus.

Tongue

The avian tongue is not composed of overlapping muscle layers, as in mammals. It is mobilized by the hyoid apparatus, consisting of multiple articulating bones and their musculature. The parrots (Psittacidae) are an exception in that they have muscles in the tongue that are independent of the hyoid apparatus and permit the flexibility required for manipulating seeds.

The avian tongue is variable in length and form in a manner similar to the beak. For example, woodpeckers: tongues are long and sticky; humming birds: tongues are tubular or semitubular; penguins: can contain posterior-directed horny hooks for holding food tightly; ducks and geese: equip with filtering processes. It is usually sharply pointed in the front and has papillae to the rear. Chickens, pelicans, gamebirds, storks, ostrich adapt their tongue for swallowing the food.

The tongues are adapted for food collection: Tongues of many woodpeckers can be thrust forward several times the length of the beak to entrap the insects. The tongues of sap-sucking woodpeckers, lories and lorikeets are relatively shorter but end in fine hair-like processes for the collection of sap or nectar through capillary action.

Tongues of certain birds are adapted for the manipulation of food. Parrots, finches and crossbills have thick muscular tongues, which act as fingers. Penguins use tongue for holding slippery prey. Waterfowls use tongues and beaks to form a filtering apparatus that retains solid food particles while permitting water to leave through the sides of the bill.

Salivary Glands

Salivary glands are best developed in birds that consume dry diets, such as grasses, seeds, or insects. These are scattered in groups around the lower oral cavity, tongue, and pharynx. In chickens 7-30 ml of a mucinous saliva is secreted per day. The saliva is adequate to lubricate a bolus of food but usually is insufficient to moisten the food enough for extensive enzymatic digestion. Amylase and lipase have been reported in chicken saliva but their significance is minor. In species that consume slippery food (e.g. piscivores), the salivary glands are greatly diminished or missing. Salivary glands are large and numerous in woodpeckers and provide a sticky saliva, which aids in adhering insects.

Taste Buds

Birds generally have poorer taste acuity than mammals. This is probably due to the rapid transit of food through the mouth, lack of mastication, and relatively low saliva addition to the food. Low taste acuity is reflected in very low numbers of taste receptors: 62 in Japanese quail, 350 in parrots, compared with 9000 in humans and 17,000 in rabbits. The tongue, oral cavity, and beak of birds have a rich supply of touch receptors, and they augment the bird's relatively poor gustatory capacity with a strong tactile sense.

It can be generally concluded that birds can taste the same four primary flavours (sour, sweet, bitter, salty) as humans but with considerably less acuity. The sense of smell is not well developed in birds, with a few possible exceptions, such as the Kiwi, and some vultures and seabirds that use smell for the location of food (Healy and Guilford, 1990). Nocturnally active birds have large olfactory bulbs, but sight and touch are clearly the predominant sense used by most birds for discriminating food and nonfood items. Flowers and fruits that rely on birds for pollination and seed dispersal are not scented, unlike those that attract mammals.

Esophagus and crop

The esophagus extends from pharynx along the neck into the thoracic cavity and terminates in the proventriculus. It has a relatively greater diameter than that found in mammals in order to accommodate food that has not been reduced in size by chewing. To aid in swallowing large food items, the esophagus is expandable and is enriched with mucous glands to provide lubrication. The diameter is especially great in birds (e.g. carnivores, piscivores, and frugivores) that feed on large items and is often smallest in granivores, insectivores, and birds that crush their food. The epithelial lining is thick and cornified for protection against mechanical damage as a result of swallowing whole-foods. The thickness of this cornified layer and the size of mucous glands is greatest in granivores and herbivores (Ziswiler, 1985).

The main function of the esophagus is to pass food from the mouth to the proventriculus. The esophagus of most species also serves a storage function. This is accomplished by the extreme elasticity of the esophagus in many species, such as grebes, penguins, geese, ducks, owls, woodpeckers, gulls, and petrels. Birds are apparently not discomforted by the presence of food occluding their esophagus. The presence of a fish extending from the proventriculus to the beak is a common sight among piscivorous seabirds and may persist for an hour or more. In some species, the storage function of the esophagus is enhanced by its widening just prior to entering the thoracic cavity to give one or more clearly partitioned diverticula, known as a crop. Crops are particularly well developed in granivores and in scavengers, such as vultures (Fisher and Dater, 1961).

An enlarged esophagus or a crop provides a temporary storage area that permits a bird to forage for large amounts of food rapidly and then fly off to digest the meal in safe cover (Hainsworth and Wold, 1972; Buyse et al., 1993). A crop also permits 'tanking up' in the evening so that food can be slowly released to supply nutrients during the nighttime. In hummingbirds, the filling of a large crop by extensive foraging at dusk fuels their high metabolic rate for several hours into the night. In chickens, food stored during an evening feeding supplies about 75% of the nocturnal energy needs.

An additional function of the crop in granivores and herbivores is the provision of a moist environment where food begins to soften, permitting more efficient digestion. However, in chickens and quail, mucous glands are only present near the entrance of the crop, so most of the water needed for softening must be consumed with the meal. There are no enzymes secreted into the crop but those present in the food may provide some digestion while residing in the crop.

In the Hoatzin, the crop serves as an organ for microbial fermentation (see page No. 120 for pictorial presentation), permitting the efficient use of plant leaves containing high dietary fibre (Grajal et al., 1989).

Crop milk: The crop and the esophagus play an important role in nourishing the young of many species. In hawks, penguins, storks, pelicans, darters, gannets, cormorants, pigeons, parrots, and some waxbills and finches the crop and/or esophagus serves to store food that is later regurgitated to feed the young. In pigeons and doves (Columbidae), the crop of both sexes produces'crop milk' for feeding nestlings. The productions of crop milk have many similarities with lactation in mammals. Brooding stimulates prolactin secretion, which triggers differentiation of the crop epithelium around the sixth day of incubation. By the thirteenth day, the epithelium thickens considerably and becomes rich in blood vessels, making the crop lining reddish in colour. The epithelial cells accumulate fat and protein, and are shed into the lumen of the crop to give the milk. This holocrine secretion has a cheese-like texture, is very low in carbohydrate, and contains about 60% protein, 5% ash, and 35% fat. As in mammalian milks, the fat in crop milk is predominantly medium-chain triglycerides.

Crop milk assures a steady supply and balance of nutrients to the rapidly growing altricial chicks. The nutritional advantage afforded by the production of crop milk has been suggested as a major factor in the pandemic success of the Columbidae (Dumont, 1965; Horseman and Buntin, 1995). Crop milk is fed to the squab for about 2 weeks following hatching. Milk-laden cells are initially sloughed off only when the crop is empty, ensuring that the milk is not diluted by adult foods. As the chick matures, crop milk is fed in combination with other foods and milk-laden epithelial cells are shed only during the times of the day when parents are provisioning their young.

Male Emperor Penguins provide their newly hatched chick with a secretion produced by the desquamation of esophageal epithelial cells. The esophageal mucous glands of the Greater Flamingo produce a nutritive merocrine secretion that is regurgitated and fed to the young. This secretion also contains red pigments necessary for colouration of developing feathers.

Birds have the capacity to regurgitate food from their esophagus or crop. Regurgitation may function to reduce preflight weight to permit takeoff in heavy birds (e.g., seabirds and vultures) that eat large meals. Physical stresses, emotional stresses (capture), and noxious chemicals (crude oil) may also initiate regurgitation in some species. Emetics, such as antimony potassium tartrate, are sometimes used experimentally to induce regurgitation so that food consumption can be itemized (Poulin and Lefebvre, 1995).

Stomach

The stomach of most birds consists of two parts: the proventriculus (glandular stomach) and the gizzard (muscular stomach), which is sometimes called the ventriculus.

Proventriculus: The proventriculus secretes mucus, hydrochloric acid (HCl) and pepsin, which have much of their action in the gizzard, where the food is 'chewed' by muscular contractions. The proventriculus can serve as a storage area as well as an area for gastric digestion in some woodpeckers, hawks, cormorants, petrels, herons, gulls, terns, ostriches and emus (Degen et al., 1994). The stomach can also be a filter in which bones, hairs, and feathers are retained and often regurgitated, as in hawks and owls, while the more digestible components move into the small intestine.

The pH of the stomach contents in falconiformes (hawks, falcons, and eagles; average of 1.6) is much lower than in the strigiformes (owls; average of 2.3) (Duke et al., 1975). Falconiformes have a hydrogen ion concentration six times that of strigiformes because pH is a logarithmic function of hydrogen ion concentration. These differences are reflected in higher dry matter digestibilities in falconiformes versus strigiformes due to the more extensive corrosion of bones (ash) in the falconiformes' stomach. However, energy digestibilities are virtually identical in hawks and owls (Kirkwood, 1979).

Often one of the two (proventriculus and gizzard) organs predominates in size, depending on the diet. In many carnivores and piscivores, the proventriculus is large and the gizzard is thin-walled and weak; this is taken to the extreme in pelicans, where the gizzard is essentially absent. In granivores and herbivores, the gizzard is very muscular and dominates the proventriculus in size.

Gizzard: The gizzard of birds (e.g., carnivores, piscivores, nectarivores, and frugivores) feeding on foods that are soft and easily digested is a relatively round organ, similar in thickness and muscularity to the proventriculus. In some nectarivores and frugivores, the gizzard is only a very small diverticulum at the junction of the proventriculus and the small intestine, where soft-bodied insects are digested. In many insectivores, herbivores, and omnivores that feed on coarse food items, the gizzard is a larger and more muscular organ. The amount of muscularity is greatest in birds that consume grain and other hard seeds. The gizzard is also well developed in molluscivores and crustacivores, in order to crush shells and exoskeletons. It is less muscular in parrots (Psittacidae), which remove the hull from seeds and fragment them with their bill prior to swallowing.

Small intestine

The small intestine functions in enzymatic digestion and absorption of the end products of digestion. Across the species, the small intestine is considerably less variable in form and function compared with the more anterior organs. The small intestine consists of a duodenum, jejunum, and ileum, although these segments are not clearly demarcated in most birds. The bile and pancreatic ducts enter the duodenum.The duodenum originates from the gizzard and forms a loop around the pancreas. The duodenum ends at the point where the small intestine leaves its association with the pancreas. Posterior to the duodenal loop is the jejunum, followed by the ileum. The jejunum extends from the end of the duodenum to the vitelline diverticulum (Meckel's diverticulum), which is the remnant of the yolk sac. The ileum extends from the vitelline diverticulum to the caecal junction.

The intestinal mucosa contains villi and crypts of Lieberkuhn. Epithelial cells of the villi have about 10^5 microvilli per square millimeter on their apical surface, increasing the absorbing surface area 15-fold. The avian mucosal epithelium does not contain an equivalent of mammalian Brunner's glands, but numerous goblet cells. They secrete copious mucus, which protects the epithelium from digestive enzymes and abrasion by the digesta. The mucus is particularly thick along the anterior duodenum, where it protects the villi from the excessive acidity of the digesta leaving the gizzard.

The most variable aspects of the small intestine, among the birds, are its (1) overall length, (2) the size and shape of the villi, and (3) the degree to which microorganisms populate the ileum. These three factors are subject to some variation within a single bird, depending upon the composition of its diet. Relative to body size, the small intestine tends to be long in herbivores and granivores and relatively short in carnivores, nectarivores, and frugivores

(Herpol and van Grembergen, 1967; Ziswiler and Farner, 1972). This is because the enzymatic digestion of meat or fruit is proficient and rapid compared with the digestion of seeds or vegetation, which are rich in cell walls. The villi of carnivorous birds are well developed and finger-like than the flatter villi of herbivores, partially compensating for the decreased length of their small intestine.

In some herbivorous species, the posterior region of the small intestine is richly populated with microorganisms and may be involved in the fermentation of nutrients that have withstood digestion in the more anterior intestine. Although the ileum is rarely the major site for microbial fermentation, it may function as a transition between the digestive functions that use enzymes produced by the bird and the microbial-based digestion that occurs in the more posterior tract.

Caeca

The caeca originate from the rectum at a location immediately posterior to the junction of the small intestine and the rectum. There is a very large degree of variation in the size of caeca among species, ranging from voluminous paired caeca to a single caecum to complete absence. For those species that have them, the most common arrangement is two caeca of approximately equal length with separate openings into the rectum. The caeca are highly developed in herbivores and omnivores, where they serve as a site for microbial fermentation of complex carbohydrates that resist digestion in the small intestine. In some species they may serve water- and nitrogen-absorption or immunosurveillance functions. Within closely related species, the size of the caeca often correlates with the diet type (Table 1).

Table 1.   Functions of the avian caeca

Sl. No	Caecal (important) function	Examples
1	Water resorption	Owl
2	Fibre digestion	Ostrich
		Many ducks and geese
3	Water resorption and fibre digestion	Chicken, turkey, quail, guinea fowl, ptarmigan, emu, ducks and geese
4	Nitrogen homeostasis	All species with caeca
5	Immunosurveillance of posterior regions of G. I Tract	All species with caeca
6	None, caeca are absent or residual (caecal functions are carried out by other organs - kidneys and rectum)	Hawks, parrots, woodpeckers, swifts, hummingbirds, passerines

Classification of caeca: Various classification schemes have been used for the avian caeca. When a combination of size and histological criteria are used, caeca can be divided into four general types: intestinal; glandular; lymphoepithelial; and vestigial.

Intestinal caeca: Intestinal caeca are well developed and histologically similar to the intestines (e.g., some species of ducks, geese, grebes, and ratites). In some species they are relatively large, and rich in lymphoid tissue (e.g. many Galliformes, such as chickens, turkeys, and quail). Herbivorous birds, such as ratites, screamers, tinamou, and many species of grouse, have large caeca that are highly sacculated or have spiral out-pouches, which provide an area for microbial fermentation (Bezuidenhout, 1993).

Glandular caeca: Glandular caeca are usually long and have conspicuous goblet cells and secretory glands in the epithelium (e.g. owls). The function of this type of caeca appears to be related to water absorption and nitrogen excretion.

Lymphoepithelial caeca: Lymphoepithelial caeca are found in Passeriformes and some species of doves and pigeons. These caeca are usually small, have negligible fermentation function, and serve as a secondary lymphoid tissue involved in immunosurveillance of the ileum and rectum.

Vestigial caeca: Vestigial (or absent) caeca are found in penguins, petrels, hawks, parrots, lorikeets, woodpeckers, swifts, hummingbirds, and many doves and pigeons. Upon histological examination, a nodule of lymphatic tissue is commonly seen within the wall of the anterior rectum, but no distinct caeca are visible macroscopically. More than two-thirds of all species of birds either lack caeca completely or their caeca are very small and lymphoepithelial.

Rectum

The length of intestine between the ileocaecal junction and the cloaca is called the rectum. A frequently used synonym for the avian rectum is 'colon'.

Cloaca

The rectum empties into the cloaca, which has a much larger diameter than the rectum. The cloaca serves as a storage area for urine and faeces and it receives the ureters and the exit ducts of the reproductive system.

The bursa of Fabricius is a prominent diverticulum of the dorsal cloaca. It serves as location for the differentiation of B lymphocytes in the immature chick and becomes a secondary lymphoid organ involved in immunosurveillance of the lower gastrointestinal tract later in life.

Accessory organs

The liver, gallbladder, and pancreas are important accessory organs of the digestive system. The liver has two primary lobes and is usually larger in piscivores and insectivores than in florivores. The colour of liver changes from yellow at hatching to dark red over the next two weeks but becomes yellowish again in laying hens. The primary nutritional role of the liver is metabolism of absorbed nutrients and the production of bile acids and bile salts.

Among a limited sample of wild birds, chenodeoxycholic acid is the predominant bile acid, except among faunivores, where cholic and allocholic acids are more common. β-Phocacholic acid is a major component in the bile of ducks, geese, and flamingos. Bile acids are usually conjugated to taurine, but glycine conjugation occurs in some species. Bile salts, along with cholesterol and phospholipids, are secreted into the bile canaliculi and collected by the bile ducts. Depending on the species, the duct from the right side of the liver may enlarge into or branch into a gallbladder.

In some species, a gallbladder is absent (e.g., Ostrich, hummingbirds, and many species of passerines, doves, pigeons, and parrots). In ducks, bile from the left side of the liver can reach the gallbladder through a common sinus. In the chicken, bile from the left duct drains directly into the duodenum without being stored in the gallbladder. The location of the entrance for the bile ducts into the duodenum varies among species. In pigeons, one bile duct enters the anterior duodenal loop and the second enters in the posterior duodenum (Crompton and Nesheim, 1972; Sturkie, 1976; Hagey et al., 1990, 1994).

The pancreas lies within the duodenal loop. The digestive enzymes produced are collected into one, two or three ducts that enter the duodenum, usually near the entrance of the bile duct. Avian pancreatic juice contains enzymes similar to those of mammals, including amylase, lipases, trypsin, chymotrypsin, carboxypeptidases A, B, and C, deoxyribonucleases, ribonucleases, and elastases. The pancreas also produces bicarbonate (HCO_3), which buffers the intestinal pH.

Digestion of Food in the Birds

Retrograde movement of digesta: The uptake of nutrients is dependent on their prehension, digestion and absorption from the gastrointestinal tract and requires the coordinated effort of all digestive organs. As the digesta moves from mouth, esophagus, stomach, intestines, towards vent, the food is denatured and hydrolyzed. This posterior flow of digesta is often interrupted in birds by reflexes in the opposite direction, which is known as retrograde flow. Retrograde movement of digesta occurs between the proventriculus and the gizzard, the small intestine and the gizzard and the rectum, the caeca and the cloaca and the rectum.

Two types of digestion may occur: (1) Autoenzymatic digestion is due to the action of enzymes of bird origin, which are produced in the proventriculus, small intestine, pancreas, and possibly other organs of the digestive tract. (2) Alloenzymztic digestion is due to enzymes of microbial origin (fermentative digestion), usually in the lumen of caeca or rectum. It is now recognized that digestion in birds involves the movement of digesta back and forth between the stomach and small intestine, one cannot use the mere presence of an enzyme in stomach contents as an indicator of its origin. The reversible flow of digesta between the stomach and small intestine in birds maximizes digestive efficiency while minimizing intestinal weight and length.

Mammals

Carnivores, Herbivores and Omnivores

In general the dimensions of gastrointestinal tract are variable as per the dietary habits. In carnivores, the gross structure of gastrointestinal tract is relatively short and simple since digestion is mainly enzymatic and microbial digestion is minimal. Domesticated herbivores-ruminants (pregastric fermentation) and horses (postgastric fermentation) have voluminous digestive tract to accommodate microbial fermentation. In omnivores both enzymatic and postgastric fermentation are of importance and have intermediate structure.

Gastrointestinal Tract

Buccal Cavity

The buccal cavity is the first structure of the generalized digestive tract. Major differences between species occur in the teeth and lips of mammals, and tongues, tastebuds, and saliva of mammals. For the higher animals, nourishment involves the prehension of food, as well as its digesion within the animal's digestive tract. Prehension is the act of taking food into the organism. Mammalian teeth are particularly important in the prehension of food and in reducing particle size for swallowing and digestion.

Mastication

In carnivores and omnivores the jaw movements are mainly in a vertical plane and produce a shearing action. However, coarse plant food/forage requires for more mechanical grinding and hence, in herbivores there is considerable lateral movement of the jaws. The upper jaw is wider than the lower jaw, and mastication occurs only on one side at a time. Because of this lateral movement, the teeth wear with chisel shaped grinding surfaces. The sharp edge of the lower teeth is innermost, and that of the upper teeth is outermost. The oblique tables of the teeth of herbivores are composed of substances of different degrees of hardness, and the grinding efficiency of the tables is increased by their uneven wear.

Digestion is preceded by the physical breaking up in the mouth into pieces leading to bolus formation for easy swallowing. The breaking up of food is called 'comminution'. In non-ruminants this occurs during prehension and bolus formation and in ruminant animals it takes place during prehension, bolus formation and rumination.

Functions and Quantity of Saliva

Saliva's major roles include lubricating food for swallowing, providing nutrients and buffers for foregut fermentation in many herbivores, solubilizing water-soluble food components for tasting, and initiating digestion through salivary enzymes. Many mammals (e.g., humans, laboratory rats, bears, moose, and mule deer) that are adapted for consuming tannin-containing foods secrete tannin-binding salivary proteins. Free tannins can impede digestion and can be toxic. Hence, these animals synthesize salivary proteins with a high tannin-binding affinity that neutralizes tannins as they are ingested (Robbins et al., 1991).

Saliva is produced primarily by the parotid, mandibular, and sublingual glands. Quantity varies with the species. Carnivores secret little saliva since they ingest slippery aquatic food or those that do little chewing because they ingest relatively moist food in large chunks. Ruminant and nonruminant herbivores secret large volumes of saliva, as they ingest drier fibrous feeds that needs both mastication and lubrication.

Salivary Enzymes

Salivary amylase: Amylase occurs widely in herbivorous and omnivorous mammals saliva but is absent from strict carnivores, such as cats (Vonk and Western, 1984). Taste and, consequently, food selection may be affected by salivary amylase as it hydrolyzes starch and glycogen to maltose and small oligosaccharides. Salivary amylase is inactivated by the acidity of the mammalian glandular stomach. But the enzyme can remain active in food boluses as the interior portion is not immediately exposed to stomach acidity and in the more neutral pH of non-glandular stomach compartments of many herbivorous mammals (Karn and Malacinski, 1978).

Salivary lipase and gastric lipase: Lipases are the predominant enzymes for the digestion of milk fat. Although fat digestion in adult animals is primarily by pancreatic and small intestine lipases, the activities of these enzymes are very low in nursing animals. The low levels of the normal, adult lipases in nursing mammals contrasts with the very high levels of fat in the milk of most wild animals (about 49% of the dry matter of mature marsupial milk, 30% for primates, 45% for lagomorphs, 39% for rodents and terrestrial carnivores, 79% for seals and sea lions, 38% for artiodactyls, and a low of 7% for perissodactyls). Consequently, fat digestion in the newborn occurs in the stomach where the milk clot entraps both milk lipids and salivary lipase (Hamosh, 1979).

Esophagus

The esophagus conducts food from the mouth to the stomach.

Stomach

Four Chambers of the Ruminant Stomach

The four chambers of the ruminant stomach are the rumen, reticulum, omasum, and abomasum.

(1) The rumen is a large, thin-walled, saclike structure lined with papillae. The papillae of the rumen increase the absorptive surface area from 16 to 38 times relative to the theoretically nonpapillated rumen wall. Rumenoreticulum provides space for fermentative digestion in the ruminants. The reticulum is approximately spherical and the esophagus enters dorsomedially at the cardia. The reticulum is partially separated from the cranial sac of the rumen by the ruminoreticular fold, which even when contracted leaves a large orifice between the reticulum and the rumen. For this and other

reasons the ruminoreticulum operates as a combined functional unit despite the clear anatomical differences between these two compartments.

(2) The omasum is a finely partitioned, weirlike structure that (a) separates the highly acidic abomasal contents from the fermenting contents of the rumenoreticulum; (b) provides for the passage of smaller food particles into the abomasum while retaining less digested, larger particles in the rumenoreticulum; and (c) absorbs water and soluble food and microbial products (Prins et al., 1972).

(3) Microbial cells, small food particles, and previously nonabsorbed metabolites pass into the abomasum or true stomach, for enzymatic and acid hydrolysis.

Vertebrates do not secrete enzymes to digest plant cell wall carbohydrates. The symbiotic relationships with fibre-digesting bacteria and protozoa enable herbivores to utilize otherwise nondigestible plant fibre and yield bacterial cells, volatile fatty acids and carbon dioxide, methane and hydrogen gas. The major volatile fatty acids produced during fermentation are acetic, propionic, and butyric acids. The complete oxidation of 1 mole of glucose from cellulose yields 38 moles of high-energy ATP. Anaerobic bacteria fermenting glucose can capture only 2-6 moles of ATP (Van Soest, 1981), while the residual 32-36 moles are available to the host via oxidative metabolism of the volatile fatty acids.

Examples of animals with forestomach fermentation include the cervids; giraffes; bovids; tragulids or mouse deer; camels; peccaries and hippopotamuses; macropod marsupials, such as kangaroos and wallabies; leaf-eating monkeys, such as langurs; numerous herbivorous rodents; hyraxes; and leaf-eating tree sloths.

Forestomach Fermentation Pouches in Rodents, Marsupials and Cetaceans

Herbivorous rodents, small marsupials and cetaceans have variations. In many herbivorous rodents the forestomach fermentation pouches ranges from a single diverticulum with minimal specialization communicating directly with the true stomach. Very extensive forestomach pouches also occur in many cetaceans (whales, porpoises, and dolphins) and several small marsupials (honey possum, rufous rat-kangaroo, and long-nosed potoroo).

Volatile fatty acids occur in the contents of these sacculations. But their mere presence does not indicate that these are important fermentation sites, particularly when the diet is highly digestible without fermentation. Some of these pouches are undoubtedly analogous to the avian crop in which food storage is their primary role. However, bacterial and VFA concentrations in the forestomach of baleen whales, which can contain as much as 550 kg of food in a large fin whale, increasingly suggest that fermentation is an important digestive process in these animals (Herwig et al., 1984).

Neonatal Stomach

Reticular groove: The neonatal stomach of forestomach fermenters functions as if the animal were a simple-stomached animal. Because milk is totally digested by enzymes of the true stomach and small intestine, reticular groove provides a mechanism to pass milk directly from the esophagus into the acidic stomach. The reticular groove is a bilipped channel passing along the reticulum wall from the esophageal orifice to the omasal orifice. As milk passes down the esophagus, the lips of the groove close reflexively to form a rumen-reticulum bypass, which continues to function as long as milk is ingested. The groove will close even when milk is consumed from a bucket (Matthews and Kilgour, 1980). This kind of a bypass does not occur in rodents and hyraxes because of the close juxtaposition of the esophageal opening to the acidic stomach (Kinnear et al., 1979; Leon, 1980).

Gastric sulcus (groove): Although a gastric sulcus (groove) occurs in some macropod marsupials, it is absent in others, a milk bypass is apparently unnecessary in very young marsupials as the stomach is undifferentiated and has a classical acid proteolysis throughout. Once the young leave the pouch and begin ingesting forage and developing areas of fermentation, the gastric sulcus may become important as a milk bypass mechanism (Hume, 1982).

Development of Rumen

Rumen development is dependent on the ingestion and fermentation of plant matter. Bacterial inoculation of the rumen is routine with suitable bacteria potentially being transmitted in maternal saliva during licking of the neonate by the mother and on maternal faeces touched or consumed by the neonate. Young deer and elk removed from the mother 6-18 hr after birth and raised in isolation develop normally functioning rumens.

Provision of creep feed to the young around 10 days of age initiates the young ruminant into solid feed. Papillary growth is stimulated by the metabolic products of fermentation, particularly volatile fatty acids. Butyrate, because of its metabolism by the rumen epithelium, provides the greatest stimulant to papillary growth, followed by propionate and acetate. Reduced milk intake increases the rate of rumen development by stimulating dry-feed intake and therefore fermentation.

Fluid from the rumen or the forestomach of marsupials contains from 11 to 760 billion bacteria per milliliter (McBee et al., 1969; Pearson, 1969; Hume, 1982). These bacteria secrete cellulase into an immediately adjacent, extracellular zone to digest plant cell wall carbohydrates. Monosaccharides are absorbed by the bacteria and metabolized to volatile fatty acids, 50 to 80% of which is acetic acid. Volatile fatty acids absorbed from the forestomach account for 21-75% of the digestible energy intake in ruminants and macropod marsupials.

pH of the Forestomach

The pH of the forestomach contents is dependent on the balance between the production of volatile fatty acids, their rate of absorption or outflow, salivary buffering capacity, and the completeness of separation between the forestomach and the true stomach. For example, rumen pH in red deer decreased from 6.5 prior to feeding to 5.5 ninety minutes after feeding when the rate of acid production exceeded buffering and absorption capacities (Maloiy et al., 1968). Forestomach pH has generally varied from 5.4 to 6.9 in wild ruminants, macropod marsupials, and hippopotamuses.

Mammalian Abomasum

Acidic Digestion

Acidic digestion occurs in the abomasum of mammals. Many carnivores are well known for their rapid ingestion of very large quantities of food that require many hours of digestion. The pH of pure gastric acid in both birds and mammals ranges from 0.2 to 1.2 (Ziswiler and Farner, 1972). However, the observed pH of the stomatch contents generally ranges from 1.0 to 3.0 in birds and from 1.6 to 4.0 in mammals. The higher pH of stomach contents than of pure gastric acid is due to the dilution and neutralization by food or ingested fluids, the internal regulation or optimization of gastric pH, and, in some species, the retrograde flow (Page No. 130) of more alkaline small-intestinal contents into the stomach (LePrince et al., 1979).

Enzymes of the Stomach

Digestion in the acidic stomach is primarily proteolysis. Pepsin is the primary gastric proteolytic enzyme occurring in both mammals and birds. Pepsin occurs in the abomasum, proventriculus, and, possibly, the gizzard mucosa in an inactive form called pepsinogen. When pepsinogen is secreted into the gastric lumen in the presence of hydrochloric acid at a pH below 5, a low-molecular-weight polypeptide is cleaved to form active pepsin. Below pH 4, the conversion of pepsinogen to pepsin is catalyzed by pepsin; thus, the reaction is autocatalytic. Pepsin activity is generally strongest between pH 1 and 2, although a second peak may occur between pH 3.5 and 4.0. The acidic environment of the stomach generally denatures ingested protein, which exposes the bonds to enzymatic hydrolysis. Pepsins preferentially split peptide bonds involving phenylalanine, tyrosine, leucine, and glutamic acid.

An additional enzyme, rennin, occurs in the gastric juice of nursing mammals and has an optimum activity at pH 4.0. Both pepsin and rennin readily coagulate milk casein in nursing animals. The digestion of the milk clot provides a continuous, prolonged flow of nutrients into the small intestine of the young animal and avoids flow surges or the excessive passage of fermentable substrates into the intestinal tract.

Chitinase, an enzyme capable of hydrolyzing the carbohydrate exoskeleton of invertebrates, occurs in the stomach of some birds and mammals. It probably occurs most commonly in those animals where insects are a significant part of the diet (Le Prince et al., 1979; Vonk and Western, 1984). Gastric lipase also occurs in some animals (Abrams et al., 1988).

Small Intestine

Length and volume: Dietary habits determine the length and volume. The length of all intestinal segments in both mammals and birds relative to body weight are longest in herbivores, intermediate in granivores and frugivores, and shortest in carnivores and insectivores. Relative intestinal length, weight, and volume within each species vary with sex, age, seasonal food habits, and level of intake as determined by changing requirements or food quality.

Secretions Entering Small Intestine

The small intestine is the primary site of enzymatic digestion and absorption. The mammalian small intestine is morphologically divided into a proximal duodenum looping around the pancreas, intermediate jejunum, and distal ileum. Digestive secretions enter the small intestine from the liver (bile salts: glycocholates and taurocholates), pancreas (buffering bicarbonate ion; proteases, including trypsinogen, chymotrypsinogen, and procarboxypeptidase; amylase; lipase; lecithinase; and nuclease), intestinal mucosa (primarily peptidases and saccharidases), and duodenal glands (alkaline fluid for pH regulation). The secretion of the various enzymes and buffering solutions is stimulated by the passage of stomach contents, called chime, into the duodenum. Liver and pancreas ducts carrying digestive secretions open near the duodenal - abomasal orifice in mammals and more distally in the duodenum in birds (Sklan, 1980). The initial response must be to neutralize the chime because intestinal tract contents posterior to the stomach in both birds and mammals range from 5.2 to 7.5, with a mean of approximately 6.5.

Pancreatic Proteases, Endopeptidases and Exopeptidase

The pancreatic proteases are secreted as inactive proenzymes. The proenzymes are converted to active enzymes by a series of reactions beginning with the activation of trypsinogen by enterokinase, an enzyme produced by the intestinal mucosa. Trypsin in turn activates chymotrypsinogen and procarboxypeptidase. Each pancreatic protease preferentially hydrolyzes specific peptide bonds. For example, trypsin hydrolyzes bonds involving lysine and arginine, and chymotrypsin hydrolyzes bonds involving aromatic amino acids. These enzymes are termed endopeptidases because they hydrolyze the interior peptide bonds. Carboxypeptidase is an exopeptidase that hydrolyzes peptide bonds in sequence from the end of the chain. The additional intestinal mucosal proteases complete protein digestion and produce free amino acids for absorption.

Absorption of Colostral Immunoglobulins

The absorption of colostral immunoglobulins is unique because the molecule must be absorbed intact by pinocytosis. Important mechanisms enabling the passage and absorption of intact immunoglobulins include (a) the time lag in acid and enzyme production by the neonatal stomach and small intestine and (b) the incorporation of enzyme inhibitors in maternal colostrum. Colostral immunoglobulins are relatively resistant to chymotrypsin but are destroyed by trypsin. Hence trypsin inhibitors occur in the colostrum of many species. Trypsin inhibitors protect the immunoglobulin without completely inhibiting the digestion of other milk proteins by pancreatic and intestinal proteases.

Saccharidases

Numerous saccharidases are produced by the pancreas and intestinal mucosa. These include amylase, which hydrolyzes starch and glycogen; maltase, which hydrolyzes the glucose disaccharide maltose; sucrase, which hydrolyzes the glucose-fructose disaccharide of plants; isomaltase, which hydrolyzes dextrans linked $\alpha 1, 6$; and lactase, which hydrolyzes the galactose-glucose disaccharide of milk.

Occurrence of lactase depends on the presence of lactose: The occurrence of the enzyme is related to the age of the animal and the composition of the food entering the small intestine. For example, those species in which the milk does not contain lactose normally do not produce lactase. Even though marsupial milk in its natural form contains only traces of lactose, the 'young-in-the-pouch' do produce lactase equal to that occurring in eutherian neonates, apparently because the cleavage of the galactose-rich oligo-and poly-saccharides produces a lactose unit that must be further digested (Walcott and Messer, 1980). In lactose-producing species, lactase is the first disaccharidase to develop and remains high while milk is consumed, but it subsequently falls after weaning as amylase, maltase, sucrase, and other saccharidases needed to digest the adult diet increase.

Intestinal disaccharidases in simple-stomached and forestomach-fermenters

The intestinal saccharidases reflect the carbohydrate composition of the normal ingested food because the carbohydrate composition of the food and intestinal contents are the same in animals with simple stomachs. For example, hummingbirds that pollinate flowers rich in sucrose have sucrase activities 2 to 188 times higher than several passerines that pollinate flowers in which the sugars, glucose and fructose, are in the monosaccharide form rather than the disaccharide (Martinez del Rio, 1990a, b).

However, the intestinal disaccharidases of forestomach fermenters often do not reflect food composition, but rather the carbohydrate spectra of the fermentation products. For example, although ruminants and macropod marsupials consume plant sucrose, sucrase does not occur in these animals. The ingested sucrose is readily fermented to volatile fatty acids, obviating any need for intestinal sucrase (Semenza, 1968; Kerry, 1969; Walcott and Messer, 1980).

Fat Digestion

Fat digestion is due to pancreatic lipase and emulsifying bile salts. Pancreatic lipase in simple-stomached animals preferentially hydrolyzes the 1 and 3 position fatty acids of a triglyceride to produce two free fatty acids and a 2-monoglyceride. Pancreatic lipase in forestomach fermenters can be less important than in simple-stomached animals as the microbes have often already hydrolyzed the fatty acids of ingested glycerides and fermented the glycerol component. The bile salts and hydrolyzed fats form micelles whose diameter relative to the fat droplet is reduced 100-fold and the surface area increase 10,000-fold. The micelle is the functional unit of fat absorption at the intestinal epithelium. The intestinal reabsorption of bile salts and their transport to the liver, termed the enterohepatic circulation, is important because bile salts are often secreted in excess of hepatic production.

Caecum and Large Intestine (hindgut)

Caeca are blind, intestinal diverticula usually occurring at the junction of the small and large intestine. They are usually paired in birds (caeca) and unilateral in mammals. Functional digestive caeca in mammals are largely confined to ruminant and nonruminant herbivores and frugivores.

The relative length of the large intestine is dependent on the dietary regimen of the species. For example, the length of the large intestine relative to the small intestine averages 6% in small carnivorous mammals, 33% in omnivores, and 78% in herbivores as fibre digestion, bulk, and a reduced rate of passage become more important (Barry, 1977). The perissodactyla (horses, rhinoceroses, and other odd-toed ungulates) and many other animals had developed hindgut fermentation capable of digesting plant fibre.

Table 2: Hindgut contents (wet weight) as a percentage of body weight and the energy derived from their fermentation*

Species	Contents (% body weight)	Energy (% BMR)
Predominantly foregut fermenters		
Ruminants and Macropods		
Black-tailed deer	0.5	1
Black wildebeest	0.9	5–7
Domestic sheep	1.1–4.9	5–15
Red-necked pademelon	1.3	7
Red-necked wallaby	0.5	3
Hindgut fermenters		
Birds		
Rock ptarmigan	1–3	15–24
Sharp-tailed grouse	1.4	14
Willow ptarmigan	1.2	4–19
Mammals		
Beaver	3.6	19
Cape porcupine	8	33
Domestic horse	8.2	72–77
Domestic rabbit	2–8	10–38

Elephant	10	122
Fat jird	–	22–35
Guinea pig	5	31
Laboratory rat	1.8–2.4	9
Levant vole	–	9–15
Naked mole-rat	6–8	12–59
North American porcupine	4.4	16
Rock hyrax	9.2–12.6	68–87

* Source: page 280 of Charles T. Robins (1993)

Functions

The functions of the caeca and large intestine include the fermentation of plant fibre and soluble plant or endogenous matter; the absorption of water and therefore small water-soluble nutrients, such as electrolytes, ammonia, volatile fatty acids and amino acids; and bacterial vitamin synthesis (Table 2; also see Table 1).

The large intestine and caeca work as a unit to selectively pass coarse food residues in the faeces while separating and retaining the liquids, very small food residues, and bacteria for further fermentation. For example, only 18% of the dry matter passing the ileocaecal-colic junction of rock ptarmigan entered the caeca as compared to 96% of liquid digesta (Gasaway et al., 1975). Similarly, more than 70% of the liquid-small particle phase digesta entered the caecum of white-tailed deer (Mautz, 1969).

The caeca-large intestine is an even more important site of water, nitrogen and electrolyte conservation in birds than in mammals as urine moves from the cloaca into the large intestine and caeca by antiperistalsis where digestion and reabsorption can occur (Braun and Campbell, 1989; Mead, 1989; Obst and Diamond, 1989).

11

Nutrients and their needs for Wild Animals and Birds

Basic Interactions between the Animal and its Environment

Wildlife nutritionists are primarily interested in the basic biochemical-biophysical interactions between the animal and its environment. These interactions include the nutritional requirements that all animals must acquire from their external environment. These requirements are energy, protein or amino acids, water, minerals, vitamins, and essential fatty acids. Other nutritionally related requirements must frequently be provided for captive wildlife. For example, oral health of carnivorous mammals is better if they are given bones when consuming soft diets or if they are given hard diets rather than soft diets (Vosburgh et al., 1982) and birds must have access to hard, rough objects to trim their ever-growing bills (Baer and Ullrey, 1986). Similarly, there are many chemicals in plants that are not nutrients but are toxic or reduce consumption or utilization efficiencies of required nutrients (Palo and Robbins, 1991). The nutritional ecologist must frequently understand the chemical and physiological consequences when these compounds are ingested.

I. Energy and Fatty Acids

Energy is provided by carbohydrates and fat. Carbohydrates are fibre and non-fibre carbohydrates. Mammals lack the enzymes to digest the fibre, which is compensated by fermentative digestion in herbivores with the help of microbiota residing in their gastrointestinal tract.

Energy is the capacity to do work or produce motion against a resisting force. Energy is of interest to the wildlife nutritionist since biochemical transformations, muscle contractions, nerve impulse transmissions, excretion processes, and all other active body functions require energy. Energy transformations may be described by the laws of thermodynamics. The first law is that energy can be neither created nor destroyed but merely changed in form. Thus, if a specific amount of one form of energy disappears (such as chemical energy), an equal amount of another form of energy (such as heat) must appear.

The second law of thermodynamics is that energy transformations produce heat and, therefore, increase entropy within the system. Simply stated, chemical energy transformations are not 100% efficient in the production of chemical work. Although many machines can use heat to perform work, the living cell cannot. Heat is useful only in maintaining the relatively high, constant body temperature of endotherms. Fortunately, a significant portion of the chemical energy liberated during catabolic processes can be used to synthesize other useful forms of chemical energy, particularly adenosine triphosphate (ATP).

The total amount of useful free energy and heat released when organic compounds are oxidized is independent of the speed of the reaction, but dependent only on initial and final states. Thus, a gram of glucose will yield the same amount of energy irrespective of whether it is burned in a flame or in the controlled reactions of the animal body as long as the end products, carbon dioxide and water, are the same. This is often referred to as Hess's law of constant heat summation. Hence, the measurement of chemical energy as the heat of combustion is most frequently used to evaluate animal energetics.

The degree of dietary energy use may vary from 0 to 100% depending on the completeness of digestion and oxidation. Gross energies must, therefore, be further evaluated to understand animal energetics.

Essential Fatty Acid (EFA) Requirement for Carnivores

Linoleic and alpha-linolenic acids are present in plants and animals while arachidonic acid does not occur in plants.

Many herbivorous and omnivorous animals can produce arachidonic acid from dietary linoleic acid. For these animals, arachidonic acid is not a dietary requirement as long as linoleic acid is in the diet. However, strict carnivores, such as cats, cannot convert linoleic acid to arachidonic acid and alpha-linolenic acid to eicosapentaenoic acid because the delta-5-desaturase activity is very low or absent. Thus, cats require linoleic, alpha-linolenic and arachidonic acids.

Sources: Marine vertebrates accumulate alpha-linolenic acid because it is synthesized by phytoplankton, the base of the marine food chain. The content of these fatty acids in animals is partially dependent on their total fat content. For example, oily fish, such as sardines, anchovies, and herring are much better sources of EFAs than nonoily smelt. All EFAs are easily destroyed by oxidation. Thus, foods and oils that have been stored for too long or at too high a temperature may have little EFA activity.

Deficiency of Essential Fatty Acid and Correction

Deficiencies occur most commonly in young, rapidly growing animals. Deficiencies are slower to develop in mature, nonproducing animals because of the reserves of EFAs and the lack of a requirement for growth.

1. Penguins fed dead smelt developed an EFA deficiency that was corrected by injecting maize oil into the smelt prior to feeding (Penny, 1978).
2. Two captive female cheetahs fed an animal-based diet (70% beef, 10% horse-meat, 10% donkey, and 5% intact poultry carcasses) developed symptoms of an EFA-deficiency (anestrous, dull hair coat with poor colouration, dry scaly skin with encrusted sores, and dull, staring eyes).

The EFA content (percentage of total fatty acids) of the beef and chicken was 0% gamma-linolenic, 1.5% arachidonic, and 0.2% eicosapentaenoic acids. Daily supplementation with two 500 mg tablets of fish oil and evening primrose oil containing 4% gamma-linolenic acid, 2% arachidonic, and 8.6% eicosapentaenoic acids cured all deficiency symptoms, including the 2-year anestrus period as both females produced cubs.

The deficiency may have been caused by improper or excessively long storage of the carcasses resulting in oxidation of the EFAs or failure to feed internal organs and fat (Davidson et al., 1986).

II. Protein and amino acids

Proteins (crude protein) have nitrogen content ranging from 15.7% to 18.9%, while 16% is used for its calculation as N x 6.25. Protein is a very general term encompassing a heterogeneous group of compounds having many different functions. Proteins are important constituents of animal cell walls and are active as enzymes, hormones, lipoproteins, antibodies, blood clotting factors, and carriers in active transport systems. Hence a continuous supply of dietary proteins must be available to the animal for these functions.

Amino Acids

All these proteins composed of amino acids (20-25), which are linked through peptide bonds. Amino acids include essential or indispensable amino acids (EAA) and nonessential or dispensable amino acids (NEAA).

Animals with simple stomachs and minimal fermentative capacity usually require 10 EAA: arginine, valine, histidine, isoleucine, leucine, lysine, methionine, tryptophan and threonine, which may be remembered by their first letter as follows: A.V.H.I.L.L.M.P.T.T. These are essential because of the inability or limited rate of the animal's metabolic pathways to produce certain ring structures and molecular linkages to meet the requirement for growth.

Animal with gastrointestinal fermentation (e.g. ruminants, kangaroos and wallabies, rabbits, and many rodents) have variable requirement for these EAA based on their life stage. Bacterial modification of dietary protein within the gastrointestinal tract (GIT) or the production of amino acid from other nitrogen sources such as urea, reduces or eliminates their need as dietary constituents.

Arginine and Taurine Deficiency

While deficiencies of most essential amino acids will reduce growth and reproduction, the consumption of a single arginine-free meal by cats can produce convulsions and death within one hour. Arginine deficiency is the most rapidly induced nutrient deficiency observed in any mammal (J.G.Morris, 1985). Cats require an additional sulfur amino acid, taurine. Most animals can produce taurine from methionine, cysteine, or inorganic sulfate and serine, but cats cannot. The occurrence of taurine synthesis in most animals and the lack of this ability in cats may be because taurine does not occur in plants, but is abundant in meat. Consequently, all animals except a strict carnivore must produce taurine (MacDonald et al., 1984). Taurine may also be required by very young infants of other mammals and, thus, should be included in milk replacers (Renner et al., 1989).

Wildlife can select diets based on their amino acid content. Wildlife management is getting intensified and zoological gardens increasingly use processed diets. Hence amino acid requirement of wildlife is assuming greater importance.

III. Water

Water requirements are met from three sources: free water (consumed directly), preformed water contained in food and oxidative or metabolic water. Water is lost from the body in urine, faeces, milk (in case of lactating animals), and by vapourization through lungs and skin. Preformed water may be as little as 2 to 3% of air-dried feeds in hot deserts or as much as 70% or more of animal tissue or succulent plants. Water content of skeletal muscle is 72% while adipose tissue contains 3-7% water. The same is reflected in water yield upon starving. Water-deprived animal potentially yields two to three times more on catabolism of protein tissue per unit of metabolized energy than on catabolism of body fat. However, water produced by the catabolism of proteins, as opposed to fat or carbohydrates, is partially offset by the amount of water necessary for increased nitrogen excretion (especially in mammals).

Measurements of free water intake underestimate total water requirements because of the omission of preformed and metabolic water. Many free-ranging herbivores, carnivores, frugivores, granivores, insectivores, and nectivores meet their water requirement during at least a portion of the year from preformed and metabolic water and, thus, do not need to drink water.

Estimates of preformed and metabolic water can be made from fairly detailed knowledge of food intake. Isotopes of water, such as tritium or deuterium oxide, have provided a simpler means than direct intake measurements for determining water flux or requirements in either the captive or free-ranging animal. Water consumption in Indian rhinoceros was 3.5-5.2 L/kg DM while an elephant can drink up to 200L of water per day.

Major Physiological differences between Birds and Mammals in Water Requirement

Several differences exist between birds and mammals that affect water requirements.

1. Birds have more intense metabolism and correspondingly high rates of pulmocutaneous water loss. Hence, birds generally dehydrate during flight at air temperatures above 7°C. Water loss during prolonged, nonstop migrations by birds may actually limit their flight range or require flight at moderate temperatures or high altitudes.

2. High evaporative water loss in birds is partially balanced by their reduced urinary water excretion relative to mammals. Urea excretion in mammals requires 20-40 times more water than is required to excrete a similar amount of uric acid in birds.

3. Because of their almost universal diurnal habits, birds evaporate much more water than they produce metabolically. Thus, unlike

many fossorial and nocturnal mammals, few seed-eating birds (only several small desert or salt marsh birds) are able to meet their water requirements solely from the metabolic water and the very minimal preformed water.

Effect of Water Deficiency in Wild Animals

(a) Delay in digestion, assimilation and excretion of waste products through urine.
(b) Skin gets wrinkled (detection of such dehydration can be done by specific skin pinch test i.e. tenting of the skin).
(c) Urine gets concentrated with increasing amount of urochrome causing yellow discoloration.
(d) If deficiency of water in animal is continued long then its blood tends to thicken with a rise in temperature.
(e) In severe water loss animal may die due to desiccation and classical postmortem sign includes well-demarcated collection of peach coloured urates in the corticomedullary junction of the kidney and general dehydration of whole carcass.

Adaptations to Minimize Water Needs

1. Preformed water content

Many of the field studies on water metabolism have provided an understanding of the adaptations that animals have for either minimizing their water needs or for meeting their requirements. Some such examples are mentioned below.

- Storage of dry seeds in humid burrows by desert rodents to increase their preformed water content, selection of seeds by desert rodents based on their water content, and discrimination between seeds whose water content varies by as little as 6%;
- Restriction of activity bouts to cooler parts of the day;
- Selection of microclimates that reduce thermal loading;
- Increased consumption of insects having 56 to 82% water by desert granivores and herbivores when preformed water in the normal diet decreases;
- Selection of succulent plants or plant parts;
- Production of relatively dry faeces and concentrated urine;

- Storage of heat by passively raising body temperature to restrict evaporation heat loss and reduction in basal energy expenditure and reduction in feed intake when they are water stressed.

2. Free water

Many species, including mule deer, chukars, rabbits, dorcas gazelle, bighorn sheep, elk, and pronghorn antelope living in relatively arid conditions can be very dependent on free water.

- Free ranging rabbit populations without access to free water during droughts have declined when the water content of the available vegetation dropped below approximately 50 to 60%. The reduction in water content in more nutritious forages forced rabbits to consume less nutritious, high fibre foods and contained adequate water to meet water requirement but not their energy and nitrogen requirements.
- Antelope ground squirrels and Gambel's quail, similarly, became dependent on other water resources when dietary water content dropped below 40% and 23%, respectively.

IV. Minerals: Macro elements, micro elements and ultra-trace elements

Carbon, hydrogen, oxygen, and nitrogen are usually grouped as organic constituents. Minerals are inorganic constituents. Minerals required or represented in the animal body by milligrams per gram are called macro elements (calcium, phosphorus, sodium, potassium, magnesium, chlorine, and sulfur), whereas those required in relatively small amounts are called trace elements or micro elements (iron, zinc, manganese, copper, molybdenum, iodine, selenium, cobalt, fluoride, and chromium). When animals are consuming highly purified diets and water in dust-free environments, silicon, tin, boron, bromine, cadmium, lead, lithium, vanadium, nickel, and arsenic may be necessary for proper growth and development (Nielsen, 1984; Mertz, 1986, 1987). These are called ultra-trace elements. However, the purity of the diet, water, and environment required to produce these deficiencies is so great that they do not cause practical problems for wildlife.

Minerals and their deficiencies: Deficiencies and imbalances of minerals are well recognized as important determinants of animal condition, fertility, productivity, and mortality (Underwood, 1977). Minerals are basically required for various purposes in wild mammals, whether they are free ranging or in captivity. Free ranging 'herbivorous mammals' fulfill their mineral requirement from following sources: Green forages and fodder (a very rich source); from soil (mainly loamy soil, sandy soil); source of drinking water from rivers, ponds, ditches.

Free ranging 'carnivorous mammals' get their requirement of minerals from nutrient flow through predation, through flesh, blood etc. In tropical climates, red ant, heaves and termites are often used as mineral licks by wild mammals (mainly by carnivores). Most of the information available on minerals in nutrition is on domestic and laboratory animals. The data can be used to evaluate wildlife diets as a starting point. Requirements for wildlife need to be developed.

Macro elements or macro minerals: Calcium and phosphorus

Deficiency symptoms and reasons for deficiencies or disorders

1. **Imbalance in the diet:** Calcium deficiency results in retarded growth, osteoporosis and rickets, abnormal posture and gait, transient paralysis and tetany, reduced antler growth. Excesses of dietary phosphorus associated with low or marginal dietary calcium levels produce an osteomalacia termed nutritional secondary hyperparathyroidism (NSH). NSH has been observed in captive psittacines (parrots, cockatoos, and parakeets) fed a diet of sunflower seeds, peanuts, and oats (Wallach and Flieg, 1967; Arnold et al., 1974), goldenmantled ground squirrels fed orange pulp and sunflower seeds (Rings et al., 1969), and carnivorous birds and mammals fed pure meat diets (Brambell and Mathews, 1976).

    Most seeds, fruits, meats, and fish fillets are very low in calcium and have calcium to phosphorus ratios ranging from 1:2 to 1:44. Shrimp and other crustaceans (having calcified exoskeletons) are good sources of calcium (Welinder, 1974) whereas insects with noncalcified cuticles are poor calcium sources.

2. **Dominance hierarchies and overfeeding:** Dominance hierarchies and overfeeding of heterogeneous diets to captive wildlife can also produce calcium deficiencies via food preferences in which items inadequate in calcium are preferentially consumed even though the total diet offered is adequate.

    For example, one of the two captive tigers offered a balanced diet became lethargic, alopecic, and anorectic while the other one remained normal. The healthy tiger ate both types of food (meat and the commercial diet). When the very empathetic but ill-informed zoo personnel reduced the meat, used it only as a treat, and thereby forced the sick tiger to consume the commercial diet, this tiger quickly recovered (S.D. Farley and C.T. Robbins, unpublished).

3. **Free ranging wildlife can also suffer from NSH.** Free-ranging wildlife consuming meat, insect, or seed diets or those animals that have very high requirements must actively seek and consume calcium supplements. Many birds ingest snails and their associated calciferous shell to help meet the calcium requirement of egg production. Lemming bones and egg shell fragments are essential sources of calcium to arctic sandpipers (MacLean, 1974) and Lapland longspurs (Seastedt and MacLean, 1977).

Similarly, adult birds that feed low-calcium fruits, seeds, meat, or insects to their nestlings must also feed calciferous grit, bones, mollusk shells, or eggshell fragments.

The consumption of fungi, insects, bones, and other rich calcium sources is essential for free-ranging squirrels, because nuts and seeds commonly consumed are inadequate in calcium (Havera, 1978).

Osteophagia or bone chewing is often observed in free-ranging mammals and is usually ascribed to a lack of calcium or phosphorus.

4. **The occasional inability of free-ranging wildlife to ingest adequate calcium** led to deficiency conditions / disorders. White-backed vulture chicks had completely normal bone formation while cape vulture chicks had broken wing bones and rickets. White-backed vultures were coexisting with large carnivores and large carnivores brought many more bone fragments to the nests than did the cape vultures nesting in the ranching area where large carnivores had been eliminated. Hence cape vulture chicks have no access to bone pieces. Meat is deficient in calcium, the nestlings depend on the adults to retrieve and feed appropriate-sized bone fragments in order to meet their calcium requirements. The adults brought larger bones and pieces of glass, plastic, china, stones, and teeth in an apparent effort to provide calcium for the growing chicks.

Calcium-deficient birds often exhibit a greater interest in bizarre objects of edible size (Joshua and Mueller, 1979). Creation of vulture "restaurants" in ranching areas where nesting cape vultures could obtain broken bones reduced the occurrence of NSH from approximately 18% of all chicks to about 2%.

Supplementation Strategies

Calcium and phosphorus deficiencies in captive wildlife can easily be corrected by the addition of bone meal, calcium phosphate, or calcium carbonate (limestone or oyster shells) to the diet, depending on the existing dietary calcium to phosphorus ratio and assuming adequate vitamin D availability. Limestone is readily eroded in the gastrointestinal tract of birds and either absorbed or excreted. Invertebrates that do not normally accumulate calcium can either be dusted with calcium salts prior to feeding or maintained on high calcium diets. Dissolved calcium in drinking water is an inadequate source of calcium, example hard water.

Sodium

Most estimates of the sodium requirements for wildlife are 0.05 to 0.4% of the dry diet. These are based entirely on domestic and laboratory animal standards. Although there has not been a thorough study of the sodium requirement of any wild animal, enough data are available to develop interspecific regressions. Minimum intake necessary for sodium balance is 9.0 mg/kg/day. Although only 20% of the sodium ingested at these low dietary levels is retained, 97% of the sodium ingested is absorbed with much of it subsequently lost in the urine. Sodium absorption in the intestinal tract occurs concurrent to water absorption and is more efficient when drier faeces are produced. The soft, more moist faeces of rabbits had 2.5 times the sodium concentration of hard faeces.

Sodium Retention Problems

Sodium retention is primarily controlled by aldosterone, a steroid hormone secreted by the adrenal cortex.

1. Aldosterone stimulates sodium absorption and retention by the kidney, sweat glands, salivary glands, and gastrointestinal mucosa. Aldosterone also stimulates potassium excretion (Muller, 1971).
2. Glucocorticoids can antagonize the sodium-retaining effects of aldosterone. Glucocorticoids are also secreted by the adrenal cortex during stress. They had pronounced effects on carbohydrate metabolism.
3. Environmental pollutants, such as crude oil, can reduce intestinal sodium absorption and thereby contribute to mortality of contaminated wildlife (Crocker et al., 1974).
4. Theoretically, sodium retention can be lessened by excessive water or potassium ingestion, since their excretion could increase urine volumes which would secondarily increase sodium excretion.

Sodium appetite is more in spring and summer seasons: Simultaneous water and potassium loading do occur when herbivores feed on lush green forages (spring season). Females need more to meet the increased demands of gestation and lactation. Hence sodium appetite is more in spring and summer seasons due to heavy loss of sodium chloride in the sweat.

Plant defenses that could reduce animal populations: The low sodium content of many plants and allelochemicals that might increase sodium excretion could be important plant defenses that would have the capability to reduce animal populations if they were unable to meet their sodium requirements (Angerbjorn and Pehrson, 1987).

Deficiencies and dietary sources: Symptoms of sodium deficiencies are reduced growth, softening of bones, corneal keratinization, gonadal inactivity, decreased plasma sodium concentration, adrenal hypertrophy, decreased fluid volume, producing shock and death.

Few terrestrial plants require sodium, and only halophytes actively concentrate it, even though this element is the sixth most abundant mineral in the earth's crust (Botkin et al., 1973). Therefore, the potential exists, particularly for herbivores, to incur sodium deficiencies.

Carnivores normally would not incur a sodium deficiency as the tissues of even sodium-stressed herbivores have a relatively high sodium content (Blair West et al., 1968). However, penguins and other marine organisms maintained in freshwater pools can develop sodium deficiency.

Productivity of marine birds can be closely linked to availability of freshwater foods: Marine birds and others feeding in highly saline lakes must purposefully seek and feed their nestlings low-sodium foods (e.g., freshwater crayfish). Although the adults feed on high-sodium foods (e.g. fiddler crabs and molluscs), high evaporative water loss and the inability to fly to freshwater can impose severe water restrictions on nestlings. Because water intake is inadequate to excrete excess sodium, nestlings can become dehydrated and die when forced to consume high-sodium foods. Thus, the productivity of marine birds can be closely linked to rainfall and the availability of freshwater foods (Johnston and Bildstein, 1990).

How free-ranging herbivores and granivores meet their sodium requirement?

Wildlife ecologists have long been interested in understanding how free-ranging herbivores and granivores meet their sodium requirement; it is also interesting to know whether low-sodium intake might regulate populations.

Herbivores such as moose, caribou in Alaska, deer in Indiana, mountain goats in British Columbia, and fox squirrels in Illinois consumed feeds having from 0.0003 to 0.0251% sodium. Soils and vegetation of alpine, mountain, and continental areas having moderate to high snow fall or rainfall are usually sodium depleted, whereas coastal and desert areas are sodium repleted.

Animals ingesting foods of minimal sodium content must either conserve sodium or augment sodium intake by actively consuming natural sodium supplements. Sodium-stressed mountain rabbits, kangaroos, and wombats excreted urine almost devoid of sodium (Blair-West et al., 1968), whereas rabbits in sodium-replete grassland and desert areas had urinary sodium concentrations 280 times higher (Scoggins et al., 1970). Sodium-stressed animals had adrenal cortex aldosterone-secreting areas up to 5 times larger than sodium-replete animals (Myers, 1967; Scoggins et al., 1970; Smith et al., 1978). However, investigators should be cautious in interpreting enlarged adrenal cortices and increased aldosterone secretion relative to sodium absorption in that aldosterone's role in increasing potassium excretion may be equally important (Christian, 1989).

Many observations of herbivores, granivores, and carnivores consuming salt or soil or water with a higher than normal sodium content, such as from mineral licks, have been reported. Elephants consume burned wood and ash in an apparent sodium drive. Mountain goats in the Olympic National Park of Washington avidly consume urine or urine-soaked ground and table salt provided by park visitors. Moose and other animals actively seek aquatic plants than terrestrial plants for want of higher sodium. Thus, although sodium is a ubiquitous element, its acquisition and retention may require extensive effort, particularly in herbivores. It may be inferred that limited availability of sodium in some areas may restrict animal distribution and productivity.

Potassium

High potassium can reduce availability and retention of sodium or magnesium

The accumulation of potassium by both aquatic and terrestrial plants has created many potassium replete-terrestrial environments. High concentrations of potassium in some plants, such as early spring grasses, can reduce the availability and retention of other elements, such as sodium or magnesium. Thus, rather than being toxic, high plant potassium may contribute secondarily to a deficiency of another element.

Deficiencies of potassium: The potassium content of growing plants and animals is usually in excess of animal requirements. Hence potassium deficiencies may be rare in wildlife. However, deficiencies could occur because of a complex of precipitating factors and should always be suspected in captive wildlife subjected to stress and prolonged diarrhoea (Newberne, 1970). Stress-induced adrenal hyperplasia and excessive potassium excretion may be the cause.

Magnesium

Magnesium is the chelated metal in chlorophyll. It is an important constituent of bone and tooth formation and for enzyme activation.

Deficiencies of magnesium: Magnesium deficiencies have been extremely rare in wildlife. One major pathological magnesium deficiency is grass tetany or grass staggers. It occurs primarily in lactating domestic cows consuming early spring forages grown on fertilized pastures. Such a deficiency apparently occurred in captive deer grazing a heavily fertilized pasture. Free-ranging pheasants apparently even avoided consuming grit high in magnesium during egg production (Kopischke, 1966).

Struvite calculi: Magnesium is non-toxic at normal dietary concentrations. But it frequently occurs in renal, urethra, or bladder calculi as magnesium ammonium phosphate (Struvite) that can be very dangerous if urine flow is impeded (Clark et al., 1982; Nelson, 1983). Since struvite crystallizes in alkaline solutions, urine acidification with various food additives (e.g., phosphoric acid) prevents these calculi (Edfors et al., 1989).

Chloride

Chloride is the principal anion of body fluids.

Sulphur

Sulphur is primarily a constituent of the sulfur-containing amino acids (cystine, cysteine, and methionine), with much smaller amounts in biotin, thiamine (two B-complex vitamins), and the hormone insulin. Thus, a deficiency of sulfur is synonymous with a deficiency of the sulfur-containing metabolites, particularly the amino acids, and is usually not viewed as a simple deficiency of inorganic sulfur.

Trace Elements or Micro Minerals

Trace elements act primarily as catalysts in cellular enzyme systems.

Iron

Iron content of the milk of domestic ungulates is very low (0.2 to 0.5µg iron/ml). The iron content of milk is usually highest in very early lactation and decreases as lactation progresses.

Iron content of milk of wild animals: Milk of wild equids has 2 to 13 times more iron than milk of domestic horse. Similarly, milk of wild ruminants can have 15 times more iron than cow's milk. Iron content of milk of pigs, rabbit, rat, dog, cat and quokka (marsupial), respectively, are 1 to 3 µg, 2 to 4 µg, 4 to 5 µg, 5 to 10 µg, 3 µg and 22 µg /ml.

Deficiency of iron: Iron is important in the development of the growing neonate's haemoglobin, myoglobin, and iron-containing enzymes. Iron deficiencies are relatively common in zoological gardens, particularly in young, bottle-raised animals (Wallach, 1970; Flieg, 1973). If prenatal liver-storage of iron is inadequate to meet all needs while the neonate is solely dependent on milk, iron deficiency is sure to occur. The main deficiency symptom in all wild mammals is anaemia. Iron supplements must be added directly to the milk or injected into the neonate to prevent iron deficiency.

Geophagia, or soil consumption: Geophagia is commonly observed in wildlife and has been suggested as an important means of meeting trace element requirements, including iron. Approximately 80% of the iron ingested by pronghorns and black-tailed jackrabbits comes from soil ingestion. It appears that the minerals of ingested soil be nutritionally important.

However, clay particles present in the soil can also effectively chelate metal ions and prevent their absorption. Thus, mineral analyses of soils can be misleading relative to their nutritional interpretation if not combined with availability measurements. Geophagia can be either a useful source of iron or a contributing factor to anaemia in wild animals, depending on soil iron content and chelating capacity of soil clay (Underwood, 1977).

Iron toxicity: Iron toxicity (haemosiderosis and haemochromatosis) is a common problem in many zoo animals. Iron balance is normally regulated by controlling iron absorption. Only a very small fraction (1 to 20%) of dietary iron is absorbed. However, damage of liver, heart and intestines can occur when iron absorption exceeds the body's need and the necessary excretion. The cause of iron overload in zoo animals currently is not understood, although excess dietary iron is suspect.

Iodine

Iodine is not required by plants.

Iodine deficiencies in captive wildlife: Iodine deficiencies in the form of both simple and congenital goiters occur frequently in captive wildlife because many natural foods, particularly red meats, freshwater fish, fruits, nuts, and seeds are iodine deficient. Iodine deficiencies commonly occur in carnivores fed unsupplemented fresh beef or freshwater fish. Thyroid gland of mammals is very rich source of iodine for a carnivore.

Goitrogenic compounds (such as nitrates and thiocyanates) present in plants competitively inhibit iodine transport. Thus iodine deficiencies can also be produced by plants with goitrogenic compounds. Examples include cabbage, rape, kale, brussel sprouts, broccoli, cauliflower, turnips, and soybeans.

Iodine supplementation: Marine plants and animals and iodised salts can be very useful iodine supplements in the formulation of diets for captive wildlife. Goitrogenic plants can be fed if the diet is supplemented with additional iodine or iodine-rich foods.

Copper

Red meat is very low in copper, whereas liver (the primary storage site of absorbed copper), heart, brain, and kidney are much higher in copper. The copper content of milk varies with stage of lactation (highest in early lactation) and species, as like iron. Plant copper concentrations are dependent on soil pH and type, content and form of soil copper, concentration of other elements and organic residues, and plant species.

Deficiency of copper: Copper deficiencies have occurred in captive carnivores (Wallach, 1971), captive primates (Obeck, 1978), and captive and free-ranging herbivores. Copper deficiencies have occurred world-wide in wild ruminants (elk, red deer, fallow deer, moose, blesbok and bontebok). Deficiencies can easily occur in captive carnivores fed unsupplemented red meat diets or adequate diets that have been excessively supplemented with calcium or iron. Excessive zinc intake (by licking cages) produced a copper deficiency from a normally adequate diet.

The deficiency in nursing rhesus monkey is characterized by achromotrichia, alopecia, while in moose it causes reduced hair and hoof keratinisation. Anaemia and faded coat colour are characteristic of copper deficiencies in captive felines that were fed red meat diets supplemented with excessive calcium/excessive zinc.

Supplementation strategies: Copper deficiencies can be corrected by (1) including copper-rich foods, such as adding liver to carnivore diets, (2) supplementing the diet with copper sulfate or copper oxide, (3) injecting copper glycinate, or (4) using various forms of slow release copper administered orally.

Susceptibility to copper toxicity: Just as species vary in their requirement of copper, they also vary in their susceptibility to copper toxicity. Signs of copper toxicity include liver and kidney damage and discolouration, gastroenteritis with a greenish discoloration of intestinal contents, and death (Henderson and Winterfield, 1975). Sheep are susceptible to copper toxicity.

Zinc

Main role of zinc is in protein synthesis and enzyme system. Reduced growth and feed intake are the first signs of a zinc deficiency; other signs include parakeratosis. The estimated zinc requirement for wild mammals ranges from 10 ppm to 70 ppm in diet. Zinc deficiency in carnivores is unlikely as Zn is generally quiet available when consumed animal tissues (10 - 80 ppm in poultry, red meat and eggs). Zinc requirement of captive wild life can usually be met by feeding and watering from galvanized pails, pipes and troughs.

Selenium

Selinium deficiency has been reported in free-ranging mountain goats.

Manganese

Largest store is in bone ranging from 3.5 ppm to 9.3 ppm. Manganese is widely distributed in most seeds, forages and animal tissue. So the deficiency generally is not observed in wild animals.

V. Vitamins

Free-ranging wildlife must continually adapt their food habits to avoid diets deficient in one or more of the vitamins or precursors. Vitamins are fat-soluble and water-soluble.

Vitamin A

Efficiency of absorption and conversion of beta carotene
Vitamin A is not found in plants but does occur in animals. Beta carotene is widely distributed in plants and insects and can be hydrolysed to retinal

and subsequently to retinol in the intestinal wall and liver. The efficiency of absorption and conversion (of beta carotene to vitamin A) in herbivores, granivores, and omnivores usually varies from 10 to 50%. Carnivores normally ingest either retinol or retinyl esters from their prey and hence metabolic systems for the absorption of carotene and production of vitamin A may not exist in carnivores. Cat as true carnivore requires true vitamin A while mink, foxes and domestic dogs have capability to absorb and convert beta carotene to vitamin A. Many marine birds and mammals may be similar to the cat as their requirements can be met by vitamin A contained in marine invertebrates and other vertebrates (Kon and Thompson, 1949).

Hypervitaminosis A: Martin (1975) suggested that excesses of vitamin A are a relatively common cause of ill health and death in captive wildlife. Typical signs of hypervitaminosis A are internal haemorrhages, yellow discolouration of the liver and fat deposits, weight loss, deformed embryos and neonates, bone fractures and reduced reproductions.

Sources: Organ meats are rich sources. Liver is the primary storage site of Vitamin A and ß-carotene (provitamin A) in animals, and therefore a major dietary source in carnivores. Smaller amounts can be stored in the kidneys, body fat, lungs and adrenal glands. Pure meat diet is a poor source. Requirement for vitamin A for cats, polar bears, and perhaps other specialized carnivores is more than for other species.

Deficiency of vitamin A: Vitamin A deficiencies are far more common in captive than in free-ranging wildlife because of the feeding of inadequate diets. Captive carnivores fed exclusively on eviscerated fish or meat without liver or other internal organs, fat, cod liver oil, or synthetic sources of vitamin A are prone to deficiencies. Granivores are also prone to vitamin A deficiency. Acute vitamin A deficiencies have been reported in free-ranging wildlife. When average body reserves fell below 550 µg/liver or 17 µg/g of liver, sex organs regressed even during the normal breeding period.

Vitamin D

Utilization of Vitamin D_3 Versus Vitamin D_2

Fish, amphibians, reptiles, and birds require vitamin D_3 and cannot utilize vitamin D_2 effectively (Hay and Watson, 1977). The divergence of mammals from the other vertebrate taxa in the utilization of vitamin D_2 has been suggested as an evolutionary response in primitive mammals to being nocturnally active. While some mammals can utilize either vitamin D_2 or D_3, many (such as lion, tiger, giant panda) preferentially utilize vitamin D_3. It is at least eight times more effective than D_2 in preventing rickets in squirrel monkeys (Lehner et al., 1966). It is due to the binding capacity and transport by blood proteins.

Sources of Vitamin D

Vitamin D_2 and D_3 supplements are commercially available, although D_3 is the preferred form for all wildlife. Irradiation is probably the main source of vitamin D for most animals, but many plants contain ergosterol which becomes ergocalciferol (D_2) when irradiated. Seeds and their byproducts are practically devoid of the vitamin. Both phytoplankton and zooplankton contain vitamin D_3 and 7-dehydrocholesterol (Takeuchi et al., 1991). Thus marine fish oils, particularly liver oils, are the largest naturally occurring sources of vitamin D_3 available for supplementation. Adult, fresh, marine fish frequently have very high levels of vitamin D_3 (Keiver et al., 1988a, b). Fish that have been eviserated or frozen for too long have greatly diminished levels (Nichols et al., 1983). Few other animal products contain any significant quantity of vitamin D, with meat being virtually devoid of the vitamin. Thus, carnivores (which have no access to organ meats and fish) and granivores are most susceptible to vitamin D deficiency (Lowenstine, 1986).

Deficiency of Vitamin D in Free-ranging Animals and Captive Animals

Signs of vitamin D deficiency reflect improper or inadequate calcium metabolism. Vitamin D is normally not stored in the body of terrestrial vertebrates. Hence deficiencies can appear within days to weeks if dietary or irradiation sources are inadequate.

Species who normally raise their young in burrows or other dark places must either have moderate levels of vitamin D in their milk, or provide adequate body reserves via placental transfer prior to birth.

Ring-necked pheasants without dietary vitamin D_3 or exposure to sunlight developed rickets starting the fifth day after hatching.

Vitamin D deficiencies should be extremely rare in free-ranging animals because of irradiation and dietary intake. However, captive animals not exposed to direct sunlight or artificial ultraviolet light sources and consuming inadequate diets are very susceptible to this deficiency. Captive maternal-nursed snow leopards, cape hunting dogs, and bolivian red howler monkeys developed rickets when not allowed to exercise outside or to consume vitamin D-supplemented foods (Encke, 1962; Wallach, 1970; Ullrey, 1984). The exposure of cape hunting dogs to an artificial ultraviolet light source for only 3 min per day prevented vitamin D-deficient rickets.

Materials that prevent UV transmission: Window glass, polyurethane-fiberglass, and acrylic glass do not transmit UV light in the necessary wave bands. Similarly, normal incandescent and fluorescent lights either do not produce UV light or their glass and plastic fixtures prevent UV transmission.

Materials that are effective UV transmitters: Glass made of vinyl, cellulose triacetate, plexiglass G-UVT, and Teflon have the potential to be effective UV transmitters. Sun lamps with high UV intensity permit adequate vitamin D synthesis.

Vitamin D toxicity: Several plants contain toxic levels of 1, 25-OH-D_3-glycoside. When these plants are consumed, the carbohydrate unit is cleaved in the gastrointestinal tract and the metabolically active form of the vitamin is absorbed. Consequently, when these plants are consumed in conjunction with adequate calcium and phosphorus, the normal vitamin D feedback control at the kidney is bypassed. Hence, calcium and phosphorus absorption and deposition proceed out of control.

Of the three plants identified for their effect to produce vitamin D toxicity, two are in the Solanaceae (potato family, *Solanum malacoxylon* and *Cestrum diurnum*) and one is in the Graminae (grass family, *Trisetum flavescens*).

Free-ranging, fish-eating mammals, such as seals and dolphins, can ingest vitamin D at levels that would be toxic to other mammals. But toxicity in these animals is apparently avoided by increasing the rate of vitamin D catabolism and by passive storage in the blubber (Keiver et al., 1988a, b).

Naked mole rats live quite well without any source of vitamin D. They have evolved a very efficient vitamin D-independent calcium metabolism. However, they have retained the vitamin D-dependent system also. When captive naked mole rats are fed vitamin D-supplemented diets, they die of calcification of the kidneys (nephrocalcinosis).

Vitamin E

Sources of vitamin E

Live or fresh fish in general are very good sources of vitamin E. Many animal tissues accumulate the E vitamin, though fat reserves are normally the site of greatest storage. Protein-rich animal feeds, such as meat or fish meals, skim milk, and bone meal, and fat-extracted plant products are very poor sources.

Why do fish Become deficient in Vitamin E?

Live or fresh fish in general are very good sources of vitamin E. However, the combination of a relatively high concentration of polyunsaturated fatty acids (PUFA) in marine and coldwater fish, the frozen storage of the fish for several months before being fed, and the evisceration of the fish before freezing contribute to producing the vitamin E-deficiency. Similarly, the excessive utilization of cod liver oil and other oils (high in unsaturated fatty acids and low in vitamin E) as a vitamin A or D supplement can contribute to a vitamin E deficiency.

Factors that are responsible for this paradox: (a) the antioxidant role of vitamin E increases its requirement as PUFA enhances rancidity; (b) vitamin E in fish is oxidized and inactivated even when stored at very cold temperatures (50% loss after 6 months of storage at - 20°C); and (c) the viscera of fish are important storage sites of the vitamin (Ackman and Cormier, 1967; Helgebostad and Ender, 1973; Engelhardt and Geraci, 1978).

Deficiencies of Vitamin E in Wildlife

Vitamin E deficiencies have been observed in virtually all taxa of captive wildlife (Liu et al., 1985; Dierenfeld, 1989). This deficiency has occurred most frequently in captive and wild animals consuming fish-based diets. Free-ranging great blue herons and other fish-eating birds may be prone to vitamin E deficiencies if feeding on a restricted diet of dead, rancid fish high in polyunsaturated fatty acids (Nichols et al., 1986). Supplementing fish diets with 100 IU of vitamin E/kg of fish may offset the oxidative loss of vitamin E during storage.

Vitamin E deficiency diseases will occur when selenium intake is within normal limits. Vitamin E deficiencies have also been observed or suspected because of muscle pathology and low plasma concentrations in captive and free-ranging herbivores. Although low dietary selenium may have been a contributing factor in many of the older cases, vitamin E deficiencies can occur in herbivores when they are fed hays with low vitamin E content due to (1) harvesting when excessively mature, (2) leaching during the haying process, or (3) storing for too long period leading to oxidation of the vitamin.

Grass and forb tocopherol levels generally increase during early growth and are higher in leaves than in stems, but they normally decrease dramatically as development approaches seed maturity (Kivimae and Carpena, 1973). Reductions of vitamin E from 80 to 90% in grasses are common.

Tocopherol degradation by gastrointestinal microflora may be important when animals consume the high-grain diets often fed in captivity (Oksanen, 1973; Sorensen, 1973). Destruction of vitamin E increased from 8 to 42% as the dietary content of maize increased from 20 to 80%.

Black rhinos and elephants are very susceptible to vitamin E deficiencies in captivity. The possible reasons may be (1) the browse normally consumed by wild black rhinos is very high in vitamin E whereas grass hays that are fed in captivity had very low levels. (2) Stress and physical exercise can increase the requirement.

Dietary Supplementation Versus Parenteral Administration of Vitamin E

Dietary vitamin E is poorly absorbed. However, depleted tissues rapidly absorb the vitamin (Eskeland and Rimeslatten, 1979). But dietary supplementation usually require weeks to months to increase the plasma concentration significantly. The most common stable form used in feed supplementation has been tocopheryl acetate. The acetate ester must be hydrolysed during absorption to produce the free tocopherol.

Intra-muscular injections can increase plasma levels within minutes (Dierenfeld and Citino, 1989), although the active form of the vitamin (α-tocopherol) should be used. For carnivores, tocopherol can be injected into the prey just prior to feeding or the prey can be raised on vitamin E-supplemented diets.

A more recently developed form of the vitamin (α-tocopheryl polyethylene glycol 1000 succinate or TPGS) has been effective in quickly raising serum vitamin E levels when fed to black rhinos and elephants (Papas et al., 1989; Kirkwood et al. 1991; Papas et al., 1991)

Toxicity of vitamin E: Vitamin E is generally non-toxic with a wide safety margin. However, excessive supplementation (e.g. 550 to 10,560 IU/kg dry diet for pink-backed pelicans) can produce haemorrhaging and death by reducing blood platelets and clotting time (Nichols et al., 1989). These problems can be reversed by reducing vitamin E intake or supplementing with vitamin K, one should remember that excessive vitamin E antagonizes either the absorption or metabolism of vitamin K (Oslon, 1984).

Vitamin K

Vitamin K is ubiquitously distributed in plants and animals and it is synthesised by gastrointestinal bacteria. Free-ranging and captive wildlife consuming relatively natural diets, therefore, may never suffer a deficiency.

When is Supplementation Needed?

1. Purified diets that do not contain green plant matter, oil seed meals, or animal or fish meals should be supplemented with vitamin K.
2. Vitamin K inhibitors (rodenticide warfarin, dicoumarol found in mouldy sweet clover) can markedly increase the vitamin K requirement.
3. Prolonged use of ingestible drugs that reduce gastrointestinal microbial activity may also require supplemental vitamin K.

Water-soluble Vitamins

Water-soluble vitamin deficiencies are uncommon in free-ranging animals because of synthesis by intestinal microbes and the general availability of dietary sources. Deficiencies of thiamine and vitamin C have occurred in captive wildlife.

Thiamine

Thiamine deficiencies have been reported in numerous captive fish-eating carnivores, such as dolphins, polar bears, mink, foxes, sea lions, grebes, and gulls.

Thiamine Destruction - Thiaminase

Over 35 species of fish and shellfish contain heat-stable or heat-labile compounds that destroy their thiamine prior to its absorption or interfere with its metabolism (NRC, 1982). These compounds are collectively referred to as thiaminase. Thiaminase in fish is normally not found in the muscle but is confined in relatively large concentrations in the viscera and trimmings, including the head, skin, fins, and skeleton (Green et al., 1942).

Thiaminase is apparently sequestered in an inactive form in the living animal and stimulated or activated by death and storage (White, 1970). Thiamin destruction is virtually complete by 90 min when dead smelt are incubated at 37°C (Geraci, 1972).

Thiaminase also occurs in newly hatched chicks and in the heart and spleen of warm-blooded animals. A peregrine falcon developed a thiamine deficiency when fed newly hatched chicks, pigeon and quail muscle, beef, and chicken gizzards and hearts (Ward, 1971).

Herbivores can encounter thiaminase by ingesting bracken fern (*Pteris aquilinum*) and horsetail (*Equisetum arvense*) (Harris, 1951).

Thiaminase also can be produced by rumen bacteria when high-grain diets are consumed (Brent and Barley, 1984). Rumen-produced thiaminase can induce a thiamin deficiency even when dietary intake meets recommended standards.

Thiamine Deficiency - Fungal Diseases

Infection and nutrition are often closely related processes. Thiamine-deficient herring gulls consuming alewives were highly susceptible to the respiratory fungal disease aspergillosis (Friend and Trainer, 1969). Antifungal agents were generally ineffective in combating the disease. When the diet was supplemented with thiamine rather than the antifungal therapeutic agents, aspergillosis mortality ceased and most of the sick birds immediately recovered.

Riboflavin Deficiency

Riboflavin is not produced to any significant extent by animals. Hence must initially come from plants or microorganisms. A riboflavin deficiency was reported in a free-ranging golden eagle (Stauber, 1973), though animal tissue is a very good source of riboflavin. Deficiency might have been precipitated by the consumption of environmental toxicants that interfered with riboflavin metabolism. Riboflavin deficiencies in many captive animals (such as the ostrich) have also been noted (Wallach, 1970). While 'curled-toe paralysis' associated with riboflavin deficiency in birds is a useful diagnostic tool, it is not to be confused with the 'laterally curled toes' produced when birds are maintained simply on smooth surfaces (Wallach, 1970).

Biotin Deficiency

Biotin deficiencies can occur if the diet is high in raw egg white (due to the avidin that binds dietary biotin). Rancid fats or moulds in the diet also destroy or bind biotin.

Vitamin C

Vitamin C is virtually absent in eggs, seeds, grains, and most bacteria and protozoa. Rapid growth, stress or organochloride pesticides may increase its requirements.

Invertebrates and fish lack the synthetic capability and are thus dependent on dietary sources. Amphibians, reptiles, most birds and monotremes synthesize ascorbic acid in the kidney. Approximately one-half of the Passeriformes are unable to synthesize and hence vitamin C is dietary essential. The remaining synthesize in the liver (house sparrow, jungle myna) or in both the liver and kidney (Indian house crow and common myna).

Human beings, guinea pigs, frugivorous bats lack the enzyme L-gulunolactone oxidase that is required for the synthesis of the vitamin C. Hence vitamin C is dietary essential in these species.

12

Evolving of Nutritive Requirements of Wild Animals and Birds

Domestic animals are fed under regimens that are intended to maximize their productivity. Food-producing animals generally do not live long enough to experience the consequences such as obesity. In human nutrition and nutrition of pet animals, adequate maintenance is of paramount importance and productivity is relatively meaningless. Diets that promote obesity are regarded as undesirable because they may shorten life.

Wild animals and free-ranging domestic animals are to be considered differently. All the nutritive requirements necessary for their survival, growth and reproduction may have to be considered comprehensively. There are reports that indicate some wild herbivores may have higher requirements for the vitamins than do domesticated animals as given in NRC publications. Wild ruminants may be underfed in zoos (Dierenfeld, 1989).

Maintenance Requirements: Energy

Maintenance requirement - feeding trial approach: The nutritionist is often required to estimate energy and protein requirements of wildlife as a prelude to estimating necessary feed intake. Although the maintenance requirement is often defined as the intake at which the animal's weight remains constant, one must be careful in using weight as the only criterion since the composition of body tissue can also change. Additional productive requirements can be determined by feeding at differing levels and measuring the rate (of milk production, for example) or success (in case of reproduction) of the specific process being examined. Thus, all the requirements can be estimated by a direct feeding trial approach, although such estimates may be applicable only to the conditions in which the measurement occurred.

Captive Animals Versus Free-ranging Animals

The use of captive animal feeding trials to estimate the requirements of the free-ranging animal poses many problems. (1) The maintenance energy requirements of captive animals are often below what might be expected under free-ranging conditions because activity and thermoregulatory requirements may be minimized. (2) The captive animal rarely needs to search for food, or flee from predators.

Energy expenditure of free-ranging ducks was approximately 15% higher than the captive, nonflying bird swimming and feeding in a large pond (Owen, 1969, 1970; Wooley and Owen, 1978). Free-ranging ungulates may expend 25-100% more energy than confined animals (Osuji, 1974; Holleman et al., 1979). The expenditures by wild herbivores may be even higher in heavily grazed areas requiring extensive food searching, in areas where disturbance by humans or predators is extensive, or in severe continental climates requiring an increased thermoregulatory expenditure. Thus, the captive feeding trial approach to estimate energy requirements, while very applicable to understanding other captive animals, may not provide the type of information necessary to understand the free-ranging animal. Hence, this approach of using captive animals has been questioned.

Birds: Requirements estimated by ME intakes are commonly used for captive birds, because accurate measures of food consumption and food energy values are possible. However, these empirical estimates suffer from the disadvantage of being applicable only to the species, level of productivity, and environment circumstance in which they were determined. A factorial summation approach is advantageous for comparative avian nutrition because it permits estimation of requirements for species, environments, and processes for which no specific information is available. Budget that partition a bird's use of ME for identifiable purposes are commonly constructed by ecologists and are used to illustrate trophic and environmental interactions with an ecosystem. Ultimately, budgets based on ME must be converted into actual diets, consisting of variable amounts of individual foods.

Mammals: Time-energy Budget Analyses

"The questioning of using captive animals in feeding trials" provided the impetus to examine wildlife requirements from a very basic perspective suitable for predicting requirements under many circumstances. The general approach has been to divide whole-body maintenance and productive processes into their basic components and measure the energetic cost per unit of time. The cost per component per unit time is multiplied by its duration in the animal's daily or seasonal life and all of the individual costs are summed to estimate daily or seasonal energy requirements. For maintenance processes, this approach is known as "time-energy budget analyses" (Goldstein, 1988).

While the actual measurements of activity costs on captive animals can be very expensive, their application to free-ranging animals can be inexpensive if activity budgets are the only thing being considered. However, a large number of biotic and abiotic variables affect the animal's daily existence. Hence it became formidable to predict the total requirements.

For smaller animals that are very closely coupled to their thermal environment, a good model of thermoregulation is essential when using a 'time-energy budget analysis' to predict daily energy expenditure (Nagy, 1989).

For 'time-energy budget analyses', maintenance energy expenditure is defined as the necessary chemical energy ingested to meet basal metabolism, activity, and thermoregulation costs. The chemical energy used as fats, protein or carbohydrates are oxidized and converted to heat. The stoichiometric relationships between heat production and gas exchanges are constant for the complete oxidation of any organic compound. Therefore, the energy used in the individual maintenance processes can be determined by measuring either heat production (direct calorimetry) or gas production (indirect calorimetry).

The composition of atmospheric air is a relatively stable (20.94% oxygen, 0.03% carbon dioxide, and 79.03% nitrogen). Hence indirect calorimetry requires only the determination of the expired air volume and composition. Respired air sampling in indirect calorimetry is usually accomplished either by confining the animal (birds and small mammals) to a chamber through which atmospheric air is pumped, by placing (in case of large mammals) a face mask having a valve system for routing expired air directly into sensors or indirectly via sampling bags, or by surgically providing other gas-collecting ports, such as tracheotomies (Mautz and Fair, 1980).

The measurement of oxygen consumption and the use of appropriate energy equivalents in indirect calorimetry is a preferred method (rather than relying solely on carbon dioxide production measurements) because the energy equivalent of consumed oxygen is less variable. In free-living birds/animals, the metabolism of a dose of isotope-labeled water is typically used to estimate O_2 consumption and thus ME expenditure.

1. Basal Metabolism

Basal metabolic rates on the basis of taxonomical categories

Basal metabolic rate measurements have been popular because of the fundamental unifying nature of the concept and value to understanding the energy metabolism of diverse biological systems (Brody, 1945; Kleiber, 1961; Schmidt Nielsen, 1970). Knowledge of BMR furnishes a useful reference point when discussing daily energy requirements of captive and free-living birds/animals. Historically, basal metabolic rates of different species have been compared to an exponential function of body weight (W).

Basal metabolic rates (Y) of eutherian or placental mammals in kilocalories per day

$$Y = 70 \text{ body weight in kilograms }^{0.75}$$

The nutritional implication of this equation is that the energy requirement for basal metabolism in case of larger animal is less per unit weight than that of the smaller animal. Compare the BMR of 0.1 kg animal with 10 kg animal; a 0.1 kg mammal has a BMR of 12.4 kcal/day (124kcal/kg), whereas a 10 kg mammal has a BMR of 394 kcal/day (39.4 kcal/kg). Thus, a population of the smaller species weighing 10 kg (100x0.1kg; N = 100) would require 1240 kcal/day for basal metabolism, or over 3 times (1240÷394) the energy requirement of a population (10kg; N = 1) of the larger species with the same biomass.

A more recent compilation of basal metabolic rates for 272 species of eutherians and 46 marsupials (McNa, 1988a) provides the equations:

Eutherians: $Y = 57.2 \text{ W kg}^{0.716}$; Marsupials: $Y = 46.6 \text{ W kg}^{0.737}$

However, many of the basal metabolic rates measured for wild mammals are significantly higher or lower than predicted by these all-inclusive equations. The variation in the BMR can be lessened when data are grouped based on food habits rather than taxonomical categories.

Basal Metabolic Rates on the Basis of Food Habits

High metabolic rates frequently occur in mammals that eat foods that are highly digestible and abundant throughout the year, while low metabolic rates occur in species that eat foods that are in relatively short supply, poorly digestible, or heavily defended.

For example, vertebrate-eating carnivores, invertebrate-eating carnivores weighing-less than 100g, nut-eaters, and many grass and forb-eaters have high basal metabolic rates. Invertebrate-eating carnivores weighing-more than 100g, terrestrial and arboreal folivores, frugivores, desert seed-eaters, and large arboreal folivores have low basal metabolic rates. Similarly arboreality can lessen the predation risk and thereby reduce the necessary muscle mass and metabolic rate (McNab, 1986a).

While the predictive equations are useful in initial evaluations of energy requirements, species-specific data should always be used when available and appropriate.

Factors that affect BMR in Mammals

Basal metabolic rates are not constant for a species. The factors that affect include age, climate, daily rhythm, food habit, activity, productivity status. Some important pertinent ones are discussed here.

Hibernation: Daily and seasonal metabolic cycles are even more accentuated in species that use **torpor** (torpid or inactive condition) to conserve energy. Daily torpor occurs in many marsupials, insectivores, bats, primates, and rodents. Hibernation, dormancy, and estivation enable animals (e.g. ground squirrels, marmots, hedgehogs, bears) in predictable environments containing abundant, seasonal food supplies to stagger the accumulation and use of energy all through the year. Energy savings due to seasonal torpor relative to remaining active range from 88% in small mammals to 66% in bears (Wang and Wolowyk, 1988; Watts and Jonkel, 1988).

Factors that Affect the Basal Metabolic Rate in Birds

1. B.M.R

Expression of the BMR as per the metabolic body size is referred to as the **mass-specific BMR**. The mass-specific BMR varies with such factors as bird size, passerines and nonpasserines, time of day, body composition, nutritional status, food habit, age, season and climate. For example, the metabolic rate of birds that is in the active part of their circadian cycle averages about 20% higher than BMR, which is determined during the inactive part of the day (night time for most species).

1. On average, the BMR of birds is greater than that of similar-sized mammals, probably because the body temperature of birds is greater than that of mammals.
2. The BMR is usually higher in passerine species (480 kJ per kg metabolic body size) than in nonpasserine (308 kJ per kg metabolic body size) of similar size (Aschoff and Pohl, 1970).

3. Among nonpasserines, families associated with marine habitats have higher BMR values than those associated with other habitats, and families composed largely of nocturnal species have lower BMR values than their diurnal counterparts.

4. Body composition affects BMR, because different tissues have different rates of metabolism. High rates occur in the kidney, heart, and intestine; lower rates occur in adipose tissue and skin, and feathers are metabolically inert.

5. Species indigenous to the tropics have lower mass-specific BMR values than closely related species at temperate latitudes, in part due to the smaller liver, kidney, and heart masses afforded by a stable tropical environment.

6. Birds that feed primarily on nectar, grass, flying-insects, and vertebrates usually have high metabolic rates.

7. Seasonal differences also occur. Basal metabolic rates in many passerines are significantly higher in winter than in summer. Seasonal metabolic rates in nonpasserines either do not differ or are higher in summer than in winter.

8. The mass-specific basal metabolic rate of newly hatched birds is usually low at hatching, rises during the early rapid growth phase, and then declines to a lower adult level.

2. Activities

Animals cannot exist indefinitely under basal conditions. They must engage in additional energy-demanding activities in their day-to-day life.

(i) **Standing:** Standing is energy demanding activity for virtually all animals, except possibly members of the genus Equus which can passively lock the legs to remain upright. A more reasonable estimate of the incremental cost of standing over lying for mammals that includes very minor position changes is 20%. The cost of standing in the painted quail, bobwhite quail, chukar partridge, guinea fowl, wild turkey, and domestic chickens averages 17.2% greater than the cost of sitting.

(ii) **Terrestrial Locomotion:** These include horizontal movement, vertical movement, burrowing, flying, swimming and brachiation. Some demand more energy. Animals expend 6 kcal/kg/vertical km climbed.

(iii) **Flying:** Energy costs of flight vary with type of flight and measurement conditions. Gliding by the herring gull, grey-headed albatross, and wandering albatross costs 2.3 times the resting metabolic rate or 3.4 × BMR.

(iv) **Swimming:** Surface and submerged swimming for aquatically adapted animals are less expensive per unit distance than are flying and running for other animals (Schmidt Nielsen, 1972). Energy expenditure by captive mammals and birds swimming either on the surface or submerged at the most efficient speed averages 2.0 times the resting metabolic rate.

(v) **Brachiation:** Brachiation refers to using the arms to swing between objects as occurs in many primates. As with other forms of locomotion, the cost per unit time varies with speed, with the net cost (kcal/kg/km) being 1.5 times higher for brachiation than for normal walking by the spider monkey (Parsons and Taylor, 1977).

(vi) **Hanging motionless:** It increases the resting metabolism of the spider monkey and slow loris by 65% and is, thus, 3 times more costly than the 20% increment for standing over resting in mammals.

(vii) **Feeding:** The energetic cost of feeding is the additional expense of manipulating and ingesting food above the cost of the general activity state, such as standing or perching. The incremental cost of eating is 11% above perching in birds and 36% above standing in ruminants (C.T.Robins, 1993; average of several values).

(viii) **Miscellaneous:** Many other energy-demanding activities occur. The energy costs for grooming, fighting, playing, ruminating, sniffing, or other activities may need to be quantified depending on the needs of a particular study.

3. Thermoregulation

Birds and mammals are able to maintain a relatively high, stable body temperature by balancing heat gains with heat losses. The body temperature of birds is generally regulated between 40° and 44°C and mammals between 36° and 40° (Morowitz, 1968). In all homeotherms, a thermoregulatory cost is added to basal metabolism to estimate the cost of maintenance. Thermoregulation is a very recent field of investigation for wildlife ecologists. Many of the ideas and methods are originated in a series of papers published in 1950 (Scholander et al., 1950a,b,c).

Field Metabolic Rate

As BMR is difficult to measure in wild animals, Nagy (2005) suggested the use of field metabolic rate (FMR) for deriving energy requirement for wild animals. The FMR of 229 free-living terrestrial vertebrates (mammals and birds (endotherms) plus reptiles (ectotherms) was measured using the 'doubly labeled water' method.

$$FMR = a\ Mb^b$$

FMR: Field Metabolic Rate (kJday-1): a-intercept, Mb body mass in gram; b-is the slope of the equation.

Endotherms (mammals and birds) FMR = 8.53 $Mb^{0.676}$ (N, 174; P < 0.001; r^2 = 0.91)

Mammals FMR = 4.82 $Mb^{0.734}$ (N, 79; P < 0.001; r^2 = 0.95)

Birds FMR = 10.5 $Mb^{0.681}$ (N, 95; P < 0.0001; r^2 = 0.938)

Ectotherms (reptiles) FMR = 0.196 $Mb^{0.889}$ (N, 55; P < 0.001; r^2 = 0.945)

Daily rate of energy expenditure was as low as 0.23 kJ per day in a small reptile (Gecko), to as high as 52 500 kJ per day in a marine mammal (seal). More than 70% of the variation in log-transformed data is due to variation in body size (expressed as body mass). Much of the remaining variation is accounted for by thermal physiology, with the endothermic mammals and birds having FMRs that are 12 and 20 time higher, respectively, than FMR of equivalent-sized ectothermic reptiles.

Energy Requirements for Maintenance-Mammals

A bird's calculated or measured BMR does not equal its daily basal requirement for dietary ME, because BMR measurements are determined in fasted birds. Daily energy expenditure for maintenance consists of BMR + activity + thermoregulation + heat increment of feeding.

Captive Eutherians

Daily energy expenditures of captive insectivores and rodents have frequently been measured at a standardized ambient temperature of 20°C (French et al., 1976). Daily metabolic rates (kcal/day) at this temperature average:

For insectivores, 66.9$X_{kg}^{0.43}$ [i.e., 2 × BMR]

For rodents of 0.007 to 9.2 kg, 85.6$X_{kg}^{0.54}$ [i.e., 2.8 to 1.1 × BMR]

For other captive eutherians ranging in size from weasels to moose,

141.4$X_{kg}^{0.75}$ (N = 14, R^2 = 0.99), or approximately 2.0 × BMR

Free-ranging Eutherians

Free-ranging terrestrial eutherians that are not actively breeding or lactating have daily energy expenditures of 2.3 × BMR, or approximately 15% higher than captive eutherians.

Free-ranging Marsupials

The slope of the BMR and daily energy expenditure equations differ in marsupials. Small, insectivorous marsupials expend energy at 6.3 ± 0.7 × BMR whereas larger, herbivorous marsupials operate at 2.5 ± 0.7 × BMR.

The energy expenditure for food-searching activities is determined by the cost of different search efforts: prey density, distribution, and energy content and the efficiency and success rate of capture. Larger predators should use less energy-consuming search methods than should smaller predators if the efficiency of capture and prey size are similar.

Energy Requirements for Maintenance-birds

Captive birds: Energy expenditure by captive birds at an ambient temperature of 30°C is 31% higher than basal metabolism for passerines and 26% higher for nonpasserines (Kendeigh, 1970). At an ambient temperature of 0°C, energy expenditure of captive birds ranges from 3.2 × BMR for a 10 g passerine to 1.6 × BMR for a 5 kg nonpasserine. At this colder temperature, small birds have a much higher thermoregulatory demand than do larger birds.

Free-ranging Birds

Free-living birds must forage for food, travel to overnight roosts, and thermoregulate. Birds that search and forage during flight expend from 16 to 38% more energy than more sedentary feeders (Williams, 1988). For these birds, the maintenance requirement averages about 2.8 and 2.5 times the basal requirement for passerines and nonpasserines, respectively (Nagy, 1987). Sea birds that live in cold-water climates have maintenance energy requirements that are 70% higher than those that live in warm water. Birds that provide food to their nestlings have high maintenance requirements due to very high levels of activity required to procure and transport sufficient food for fast-growing young. During this crucial period, the parents' maintenance requirement exceeds fourfold basal requirement in many species. The extent of increase in maintenance requirements is diet-dependent. Faunivorous species must expend considerable effort (due to aggressive territorial behaviour) to procure food relative to that expended by many omnivorous, frugivorous and granivorous speices.

Protein Requirements

Estimates of protein requirements of animals are more difficult to make than estimates of energy requirements. The reasons are dietary protein use may depend on its amino acid composition, the proportion of protein to usable energy within the diet, and the amount of food consumed. In times of insufficient dietary energy, amino acid can be deaminated to meet the energy shortage.

1. Mammals

Dietary Protein Requirements in Weaned Mammals

Dietary protein requirements for maximum growth in weaned mammals range from 35% for cats, 25 to 38% for mink and foxes, 19% for rhesus monkeys, 15 to 18% for guinea pigs, voles, and hamsters, to 13 to 20% for deer and other ruminants. These requirement estimates do not apply to nursing animals as the dry matter of milk frequently has a much higher protein content. Even though the absolute protein requirement may be similar for both nursing and weaned young animals, the very high concentration of digestible energy in milk lessens total dry matter intake of nursing animals relative to the less digestible diets consumed by weaned animals. The required dietary protein content must increase as the available energy content increases because protein requirements must be met simultaneously with energy requirements.

Protein Requirements for Adults

The dietary protein requirement for maintenance of adult mammals ranges from 18 to 30% for carnivores, 8 to 10% for ground squirrels, 5 to 9% for wild ruminants, to as little as 1.4% for sugar gliders. Of all the mammals, cats and perhaps other strict carnivores have the highest protein requirement. This occurs because much of the protein in a normal meat diet is used to meet the animal's energy requirements. Consequently, liver enzymes that deaminate amino acids in cats have a very high, constant activity rate. These estimates are useful guidelines in formulating diets for captive wildlife. However, a more basic approach is necessary to understand the requirements of free-ranging wildlife.

2. Birds

Protein requirements: Protein requirements as a percentage of the diet decrease with increasing age. The very rapid weight gain during early life requires more protein than does tissue maintenance and replacement by the adult animal. For example, the requirements of galliformes decrease from as much as 30% during very early growth to 12% for adult maintenance. Adult passerines require as little as 4 to 5% dietary protein for maintenance (Martin, 1968; Izhaki and Safriel, 1989). The requirement for adult galliformes increases during egg-laying to approximately 20%. Since these requirement estimates are a qualitative description of the amount of protein necessary to supply both essential and nonessential amino acids, the actual dietary protein requirement will fluctuate depending on dietary protein quality and energy availability (NRC, 1984).

Requirements for Reproduction of Wild Mammals and Birds

1. Mammals

Wildlife reproductive characteristics and success are closely linked to feed resources. Nutrients are needed for the activity of reproductive organs. These have been worked out on measurement of energy and nutrients necessary for reproduction, including that contained in sperm, egg, foetus, enlarged reproductive organs (testes, ovary-oviduct, uterus, or mammary gland), or milk and the additional heat necessary for incubation in birds.

The reproductive requirements are additional to normal maintenance processes. Hence, maternal or paternal tissues can be mobilized to meet the immediate energy or nutrient requirements of reproduction in times of exigency. The tissue mobilization does provide a mechanism to distribute the very high cost over a much longer period of time.

Many other costs or consequences are involved in the total reproductive effort. For example, many birds and mammals do not moult while reproductive demands are high (King, 1973). Increased time and energy expenditures during food searching or territorial defense may predispose reproducing adults to higher mortality (Nur, 1988). Territorial establishment and defense, nest or burrow construction, and courtship are often additional energetic costs. Thus, the ecologist must recognize the far-reaching implications of reproductive demands.

Gestation Requirements

Mammalian gestation periods and birth weights increase as power functions of maternal weight. Birth weight is a reflection of metabolic body weight in which the larger species produce a neonate that represents an increasingly smaller proportion of adult weight.

Female gestation requirements largely depend on the amount of energy and matter retained by the gravid uterus and enlarging mammary gland and the increased maintenance costs of these structures. The foetus represents 80% of the energy retained by the gravid uterus (Robbins and Moen, 1975a). Foetal growth during gestation is a curvilinear function in which most of the increase in mass occurs after 50-60% of the gestation period has elapsed. The energy requirements and feed intake of pregnant females are from 17 to 32% higher than nonreproducing females. However, only 10 to 20% of this additional energy is retained as new tissue by the developing uterus with the rest of the energy lost as heat.

Lengthening the gestation period by slowing the growth rate will disproportionately increase the total energy cost per unit of foetus. That is why most of the delays during pregnancy occur prior to the initiation of growth (i.e. delayed fertilization or implantation) rather than slowing the growth rate of the foetus. Slowing foetal growth rate can be advantageous if dietary protein or minerals are limiting, as might occur for a frugivorous or folivorous primate because of the low available protein content of most fruit and tree leaves.

Body Composition of the Neonates

The mammalian neonate averages 12.5% protein and 2.7% ash at birth. Neonatal fat, water and energy content do vary between species. Neonatal seals, guinea pigs and humans contain 4-8 times more fat than do the other mammals, whose fat content averages 2.1%. The fat reserves of the guinea pig are catabolised during the first few days postpartum, while those of the seal are necessary because of the cold environment and short lactation. The very low fat content of most neonatal mammals occurs irrespective of whether they are precocial or altricial at birth. The white-tailed deer (precocial) is born with a well-developed hair coat and follows its mother shortly after birth. It has the same fat content as the very altricial mouse or vole. The survival times of most neonates (with low fat contents) are only a few hours to days without maternal care.

What are altricial and precocial? Species whose young are incapable of moving around on their own soon after hatching or being born are referred to altricial. Altricial young are born helpless (closed eyes are common) and require care for a specific amount of time. Species whose young are immediately or quickly mobile are known as precocial.

Lactation Requirements

Lactation is 2 to 3 times more costly than gestation. Total energy expenditure (including the milk produced) by lactating females usually ranges from 4 to 7 x BMR, or 65 to 215% higher than the nonlactating female. Larger species tend to have longer lactation periods. However, one of the shortest lactation periods occur in hood seals (179 kg maternal BW) in which the pup grows from 22 to 44 kg is only 4 days and 70% of the gain in body weight being fat.

Esophageal or Crop Secretions-'Crop Milk'

Mammals are not unique in nourishing their offspring with parental secretions, although few exceptions exist. Pigeons and doves, penguins, and flamingos feed esophageal or crop secretions to the hatchling. Because of the analogous role of these avian secretions, the pigeon is said to produce crop milk. Pigeon milk is produced by both parents and consists of sloughed, fat-loaded, epithelial cells of the crop wall. Crop milk is the only nourishment for the young pigeon during the first 3 days. Subsequently, the milk is increasingly mixed with grain until milk production stops at 3 to 4 weeks (See Page No. 124 also).

2. Requirements for Reproduction- Birds

Gamete Synthesis: The daily requirement of males for testicle growth and sperm production are quite minimal. Growth of the ovary and oviduct preparatory to egg synthesis increases the daily energy requirement by approximately 4% of BMR and the protein requirement by 28% of the maintenance level.

Egg production: Requirements for egg production are dependent on the number and size of eggs laid, their composition, and the temporal sequence of yolk and albumen synthesis. Average egg size in interspecific comparisons is inversely proportional to body weight - that is, smaller birds generally lay larger eggs relative to body weight than do larger birds. Although the number and size of eggs laid are characteristic of a species, both do vary with age of the female, time of laying, and food availability. Variation in egg composition between species largely reflects the differing stage of embryonic development at hatching (Southerland and Rahn, 1987).

Eggs of precocial and altricial birds: The eggs of precocial species have larger yolks than do eggs of altricial birds. Yolk contains virtually all of the high-energy lipids, less water, and more protein than the albumen [protein content of fresh yolk = 16.0%, albumen = 8.6%]. Hence, increasing the relative size of the yolk increases the amount of energy and protein per unit of egg available for embryonic development in precocial species.

The daily requirement for egg production can be estimated by proportioning the energy and protein content of the egg over the number of days required for its synthesis and deposition. Yolk synthesis within the ovary requires from 4 to 26 days, whereas albumen synthesis and deposition occurs during 1 to 2 days that the ova passes through the oviduct.

Energy requirements for egg production: The estimated daily energy requirement for egg laying ranges from 29% of the basal metabolic rate in hawks and owls, which lay one egg approximately every third day, to over 200% in waterfowl, which lay a relatively large, high-energy egg each day until the clutch is complete. These theoretical estimates are quite similar to measurements on individual species within these groups, such as boat-tailed grackles and house sparrows (12 to 47% of BMR), kestrel (39%), American coot (121%), and wood duck (178%).

Protein requirements for egg production: The estimated daily protein requirement increases from 72% above the maintenance requirement in hawks and owls to 220% in waterfowl, gulls, and terns. Birds meet these relatively high energy and protein requirements by reducing other non-essential costs, accumulating fat prior to laying, mobilizing fat reserves as well as some protein from internal organs or muscles during laying, increasing feed intake, or altering the diet to include more nutritious foods, particularly insects.

Incubation

The cost of incubation is any excess heat generated to initiate and continue embryonic development within the egg above what would normally be produced by the nonincubating bird. Many of these measurements have been done in captive birds because of difficulty in measurement in free-ranging birds.

The actual cost of incubation is dependent on adult size, clutch size, quality of nest insulation, and the temperature gradient. Incubation at ambient temperatures within the bird's thermoneutral zone does not impose any additional cost, i.e., normal heat loss through the brood patch is adequate to maintain an appropriate egg temperature. During late incubation, the developing embryo also becomes an increasingly important source of heat.

Ecologically, one of the main costs of incubation for many birds is the reduced time available for feeding. Many birds have either very prolonged incubation shifts or only one parent does all of the incubation (examples petrels, penguins, or geese). In such cases, the incubating bird depends on reserves accumulated prior to nesting. Arctic nesting female Canada geese and common eiders lost 44 % of their body weight and were on minimal feeding during the incubation time. After the eggs hatched the emaciated female birds feed almost continuously to regain the weight.

Productive Costs of Wild Mammals and Birds

1. Body Growth

Growth in all animals, particularly wildlife, has both positive and negative phases. Nutrient requirements for growth are dependent on the rate and composition of the gain.

(i) **Body composition:** The major components of the ingesta-free animal body are fat, water, protein and minerals. Glucose and glycogen are the two major carbohydrates and their concentration is always less than 1.0%. Body lipids function as energy reserve, as structural elements in cell and organelle membranes, and as sterol hormones. Carbohydrates are a major energy reserve for plants while fat storage is essential for active animals since eight times more calories can be stored as fat per unit weight.

Because body composition by whole body grinding is inappropriate for many studies, hundreds of investigators have attempted to develop indirect indices of body composition or condition (Kirkpatrick, 1980). The best method to determine body composition in the living animal is tritiated (Reddy, 1981; Prasad et al., 1983) or deuterated water dilution. However, water dilution is not an instantaneous measurement. Two of the more recent techniques are bioelectrical impedance analysis (BIA) and total body electrical conductivity (TOBEC). Both the methods measure the electrical conductivity of the body and are based on the observation that the conductivity of lipids is 4 to 5% that of lean tissue, body fluids, and bone. Thus, the measure of total body conductivity can provide an estimate of body fat content. The equipment is suitable for field use and provides an estimate of body fat content within minutes.

(ii) **Growth Rates:** The maximum growth rates of young animals are apparently established by genetically determined physiological limits to cellular metabolism (Ricklefs, 1973).

- Altricial birds grow at rates twice that of similarly sized precocial birds and placental mammals.
- Precocial and altricial mammals grow at approximately the same rates. Marsupials and primates have very slow growth rates, while pinniped carnivores (California seal-lion, Harp seal, Hooded seal, etc) have very high rates relative to the adult body weight.

(iii) **Growth Requirements:** Energy requirements are a function of the chemical energy content of the different body constituents. Body water and ash have no available chemical energy (i.e., 0. kcal/g), while anhydrous body protein and fat have 5.42 kcal/g and 9.11 kcal/g, respectively, in wild birds and mammals. Consequently, the energy content of the gain or loss can range from 0 (i.e., water or minerals) to 9 kcal/g (fat) depending on the composition of the weight change.

Fat accumulation in wildlife: The caloric content of the gain during growth in wildlife increases curvilinearly, as body weight increase because of decrease in the body water content and increase in the fat content during growth. The energy requirement for growth of young animals tends to be well below the theoretical maximum of 9kcal/g because few wild animals accumulate large amounts of fat. The potential for fat accumulation in a species is an evolutionarily determined balancing process between the benefits and costs of energy storage.

The positive benefits of fat accumulation are reduced chance of starvation when feed is not available. The negative costs are maintaining and transporting the extra weight, therefore increasing the predation risk due to the reduced efficiency or speed of fleeing from predators besides the increased feed requirements. Consequently, fat accumulation is highest in species consuming feed resources that are unpredictable in their availability.

What is the reason for variability in the fat and energy content of the gain in birds and mammals?

The fat and energy content of the gain are much more variable than the protein deposition in young birds and mammals. The accumulation of fat depends on the availability of post-fledging care to the neonates and availability of food in the environment.

Young Birds

The energy content of the gain is highest in fish or plankton-feeding seabirds (marine birds: petrels, auklets, and gannets) whose parents provide no post-fledging care (Roby, 1991). Cormorants, gulls, terns, and other seabirds with extensive post-fledging parental care accumulate much smaller lipid reserves. The lowest fat accumulation and energy content of the gain occurs in granivorous and omnivorous passerines that normally have the most predictable, easiest to acquire food resource.

Among the aerial-feeding insectivorous birds, lipid storage and the energetic cost of nestling growth are highest in those species, feeding in higher aerial strata, where insect abundance is the least predictable due to weather and those species with no post-fledging parental care. Vultures that also feed on an unpredictable feed resource (i.e. dead animals) tend to accumulate moderate fat reserves during the nestling period.

The protein requirement for avian growth depends on the functional maturity of the muscles at hatching. The protein content per unit of gain is initially lower in altricial than precocial species. But growth during the later nesting stages of altricial species contains the same protein concentration as in precocial birds.

Young mammals (Examples for comparison are seals, brown lemming and deer, mice, and voles)

The energy content of growth in young mammals is highest in seals, intermediate in the brown lemming, and least in deer, mice, and voles.

Many newborn seals store a great deal of fat during a relatively short but extraordinarily intense lactation. Blubber accumulated during lactation is metabolised when the young seals are completely abandoned by their mothers and when they must learn to catch their own food, frequently in a relatively cold environment. Thus, the strategy of these seals in providing fat stores to the young prior to weaning process is similar to the marine birds that have no post-fledging parental care.

White-tailed deer, old-field mice, common voles, and bank voles accumulate relatively little fat during neonatal growth. Thus the energetic cost of growth ranges from 1.5 to 3.5 kcal/g.

For most tropical and temperate mammalian herbivores, granivores, and omnivores that are born during times of seasonal food abundance, the predictability of these food resources minimizes the need of extensive fat deposition.

In addition, daily and seasonal cycles of fat deposition occur in many wild animals as a prelude to times when energy intake will be less than energy expenditure, such as during daily gain-loss cycles or in preparation for migration, hibernation, or reproduction.

The protein content of growth in terrestrial mammals is similar to that occurring in altricial and precocial birds. For example, the protein content of the gain in the precocial deer starts at 20%, whereas the altricial rodents being at 16%, but both increase to 23% in the adult. The protein content of the gain actually decreased during growth in the ringed seal due to extensive fat deposition. Thus, for both young birds and mammals, the fat and energy content of the gain are much more variable than the protein deposition.

(iv) Weight loss and starvation - Three phases

Large birds and large mammals: During the long-term fasting in birds and mammals that accumulate large fat reserves, weight loss occurs in three phases.

Phase I is a relatively short period characterized by rapid weight loss, emptying of the gastrointestinal tract, very little fat loss, and primarily glycogen and protein utilization to meet energy requirements.

Phase II is a very long, constant weight loss that is much slower than in phase I. The reduced rate of weight loss is due to a shift to primarily fat utilization, reduced protein loss (protein-sparing), and energy conservation by reducing basal metabolism and activity. The duration of this phase depends on the initial body fat content as fat represents more than 80% of the energy mobilized. At the end of phase II, most of the reserve fat stores have been mobilized.

Phase III is a period of increasing protein utilization to meet energy requirements and, therefore, rapid weight loss.

The composition of the weight loss is a major determinant of the rate of weight loss, since the energy content of the weight loss can range from over 6 kcal/g when fat is the main energy reserve to as little as 2 kcal/g when protein or glycogen are used. Animals can recover from early phase III starvation, although later stages become irreversible. Animals that have starved to death will contain a small amount (0.2 to 1.3% of body weight) of nonmobilizable, structural lipids.

Small birds and mammals: For many small birds and mammals that store very little fat, the three phases of starvation either do not occur or they occur over a very short time span (hours). For example, most nonhibernating small mammals and birds can survive only one to three days of fasting. Survival times generally increase with body weight, since larger animals generally store more fat and have a lower metabolic rate per unit of weight. Hares and some grouse can survive fasting for three days to over a week.

2. Pelage and plumage

Hair and feathers are of interest to the nutritionist because of their role in thermoregulation and the need to quantify the additional nutrients necessary for their growth (termed adult growth) and replacement. The periodic replacement of pelage or plumage is called 'moult' and it can be partial or complete and can happen in various birds or mammals from one to three times per year.

Hair and feathers are primarily protein and contain 93-98% protein. The principal protein of these structures is keratin, which is high in cystine. Total feather weight in birds is of 6.3% of body weight, while hair weight in mammals is only 2.0%. Thus, the lower conductivity of birds relative to mammals is, in part, due to more insulation on birds than that in mammals.

Nutrient requirements: Moulting by birds increases their daily protein requirement from 43 to 76% above the maintenance cost. Moulting also increases energy metabolism. Moulting in penguins is a very intense process as the birds remain out of water during the entire 12 to 34 days, do not feed, and, therefore, lose from 9 to 45% of their initial body weight. The increased resting metabolism is due to the inefficiency of tissue mobilization and feather synthesis and increased thermoregulatory costs due to the reduced insulation.

3. Antlers

Dead, oven-dried antlers contain 54.0% ash, 45.0% protein, 1.0% fat, and energy of 2.53 kcal/g. Because antlers grow as much as 130 g dry matter/day in moose, large amounts of energy and matter can be accumulated in these structures. However, antler growth occurs at the time when forage resources are most abundant, and thus antlers are probably not a significant ecological cost.

4. Disease and injury

The interaction of nutrition and disease has not been investigated thoroughly in any species. Virtually all wildlife carry disease or parasitic organisms throughout life and the alterations they cause in host metabolic processes would be for far more important. In most cases, malnutrition and the course of an infectious disease act synergistically to reduce host resistance and increase the detrimental consequences. Most disease or injury processes markedly increase energy and nitrogen metabolism.

13

Feeding Habits - Feeding and Nutrition of Wild Animals

Significance of Feeding Wild Animals

Feeding of wild animals is different under captive conditions and in free-ranging conditions. Feeding is a controlled activity in case of captive wild animal species, while in case of free-ranging species the animal by itself attempt to have some control measures. Feeding habits are different in case of captive wild animal species. Hence, one should have a preliminary knowledge of the feeding related activities in the concerned wild animal species. Basic knowledge of nutrition, diet and feeding method are essential.

Significance of Balanced Feeding

Balanced feeding ensures appreciable health status, acquire good immune status, maximal infant survival rate, maximal reproduction and longer life span of the animal.

Feeding Habits of Wild Mammals

Wild mammals include carnivores, omnivores and herbivores. The feeding habit varies from species to species.

Carnivorous Animals

- The carnivores such as lions and tigers prefer larger pieces of meat to alleviate hunger more readily than the smaller meat pieces. Lions and tigers carry the beef pieces to one side of the cage before they sit for feeding.

- The posture of consumption is variable. In lion, tiger and jaguar the posture of consumption is of extending the forelegs and holding the meat while the hindlegs are tucked up within the body. But in panthers all the four legs tucked up within the body. Wild dogs eat while in standing position in a hurried gulping manner as much food as they can and finish eating their prey quickly to avoid any undue attention. The parent regurgitates the meat eaten for the pups to eat.

- Time taken to consume the meat: The large felines like tiger, lion, panther and jaguar eat in a very slow manner taking 16.5 minutes to 39 minutes.

- Almost all species of the carnivores eat quickly in winter than in summer.

- Chewing bones is a preferred activity among the lions, tigers and jaguars and the activity is less in panthers.

- Tigers soon after feeding lick the cage wall few times and then drink water, whereas lions prefer to drink water soon after feeding.

- After the weekly starvation, lions and tigers show a characteristic restlessness on hearing the sound and arrival of the food delivery vehicle.

- Tigers, jaguars and panthers show a preference for chicken meat over beef.

- See also Appendix for additional information on feeding habits.

Animal Fibre for the Gastrointestinal Health of Obligate Carnivores

It is known that plant fibre is important - soluble fibre for general well-being and insoluble fibre for gastrointestinal tract health of the living beings. In true carnivorous animals undigested (enzymatically) tissues perform similar function. The recent experimental findings in wild felids (cheetah) proved that point.

Wild felids are obligate carnivores. It is likely that poorly enzymatically digestible animal tissues determine hindgut fermentation, instead of plant fibre. Using a cross-over design, the 14 cheetahs were fed exclusively whole rabbit or supplemented beef for one month each (Depauw et al., 2013). The faecal concentrations of short-chain fatty acids (SCFA, including branched-chain fatty acids, BCFA), indole and phenol were measured. Total BCFA and putrefactive indole and phenol were lower in cheetahs that were fed whole rabbit. Additionally, decreased concentration of serum indoxyl sulphate (a toxic metabolite of indole) was observed in the cheetahs fed whole rabbits. The decrease in putrefaction when fed whole rabbits could be caused by the presence of undigested tissue, such as skin, bone and cartilage that might have fibre-like functions.

Herbivorous Animals

- Elephants use trunk as prehensile organ, the grass materials may be striked on its own legs to wither away the dirt or sand and then by using the trunk, they may place the feed materials into the mouth. The trunk will not be protruded during eating activities of the elephant.
- Bears have the habit of climbing the trees or rocks in order to remove the bee-hives and by using forelimbs, the hives are destroyed and use to suck honey in addition to lapping using tongue.

Dry Matter Intake (DMI) of Wild Mammals

DMI of certain mammals is as follows - wild buffalo 1.6 - 1.7% of body weight (BW), wild sheep 1.7 - 4.8% BW, wild goat 1.5 - 5.9 % BW and elephant 1.4 - 1.6% BW. In male and female giraffes, it is 1.6 and 2.1% BW, respectively. The DMI in black buck based on the type of green fodder is as follows - 2.2 -3.5% BW on oats and berseem fodder; 2.2% BW on maize fodder.

Feeding and Nutrition of Elephants

Feeding behaviour

Asiatic elephants (*Elephas maximus*) are categorized as an endangered species by IUCN. Elephants are the largest terrestrial mammals. They are mixed feeders preferring grasses, yet consuming leaves, branches and bark of trees (Alaxender, 1975). Water is an important part of their diet. The peak feeding hours are in early mornings and late afternoons. Elephants spend most of the day preparing and eating their feed as they have to consume large quantities mainly for two reasons: large size (as adult weighs up to 4000-5000 kg) and poor feed utilization. Adults are reported to spend 18-20 hrs daily in the feeding activity itself. They sleep just for 2-4 hours and they frequently go for drinking water during most of the night and mid day.

Feeding of elephants in captivity: In India, there are various systems of keeping elephants in captivity. These systems can be grouped mainly into three categories: Intensive system, extensive system and the system followed in zoos/circuses.

Intensive system: The intensive system of feeding is followed mainly where the elephants are kept more or less individually e.g. by private owners (temples, big landlords) and the state elephants. In this system, elephants are fed exclusively on prepared feeds and fodder.

Extensive system: It includes the working elephants maintained in the jungle villages. In this system, the animals are left in the nearby forest for their feed during the period of rest. In some places supplemental feeding consisting of millet, rice, copra, sugarcane and salt is also practiced.

Nutrient Requirements and Feeding of Elephants

Elephants are classed as mega herbivores. Nutrient requirements are not known. These are fed empirically based on the experiences of Mahouts. In principle roughage based diet with little or no supplement should be adequate for an adult elephant. Dry matter intake varies from 1to 1.5% body weight in adults and up to 2% or more in young elephants. In most of the National parks, adult elephants are supplemented with various proportions of cereals, pulses and byproducts. The amounts of concentrate being fed to elephants vary from place to place and most of the captive elephants in India are fed with 5-14 kg of concentrates (Arora, 2001).

Optimum level of concentrate supplementation: Elephants are prone to obesity and excessive feeding of concentrates would aggravate the problem. On the other hand, insufficient levels may cause deficiency of one or more nutrients. Improper feeding may also lead to chronic foot lesion and other health related problems. Therefore, it is necessary to know the optimum level of concentrates in the diet of Asiatic elephants and sub-adult elephants
Asiatic elephants of 14-52 years age (1909-3968 kg BW) were used in the feeding trials (Das et el., 2012). All the elephants were allowed to forage in the nearby forests for 6 h per day and to take bathe in the natural stream for 2h/d. They were fed on cut tree fodder (*Rohini, Mallotus philippensis*) *ad libitum* during the time in their night shelter. The concentrate supplement, wheat roti was offered at 0.06, 012 or 0.18% of body weight in the three trials. Feed consumption was not significantly different among the groups. It was concluded that the amount of wheat-roti should be restricted to 0.06% of body weight in the diet of semi-captive Asiatic elephants when they had free access to forages. Enhanced wheat-roti increased the blood glucose

concentration and may cause obesity. It was also found that adult animals need 139.9 kcal DE per kg metabolic body weight as maintenance requirement.

Shrikant Katole et al (2012) conducted a study in sub-adult (7-12 years of age) elephants in Dudhwa National Park, Lakhipur Kheeri, Assam. *Arundo donox, narkul* grass (7.5 to 9.5 % CP) was offered ad *libitum*. Wheat-roti supplement or rice-lentils supplement was offered to the three animals in each group. Dry matter consumption was not different between the two groups. Digestibility and nutrient utilization data revealed that rice-lentil (11.5% CP) was better compared to wheat-roti (20.1% CP).

Feeding and Nutrition of Hippopotamus

The family Hippopotamidae includes two genera: *Choeropsis liberiensis* (Pigmy hippopotamus) and *Hippopotamus amphibious* (Hippopotamus). The Hippopotamus are the second largest land animals, first being the elephants.

The hippo is an unusual animal. The day time activities are restricted in water and night time on the land. This resulted in a unique skin structure which causes a high water loss when the animal is in the air and therefore, makes it necessary for the hippo to live in water during the day. The sebaceous gland is absent in hippos. The pigmy hippopotamus resembles a young hippopotamus in size. It is less aquatic than the hippopotamus. Hippopotamus are born, nurse, grown up, mate and spend most of their life in water. Weight of young one at birth is 42kg.

Feeding behaviour: The hippopotamus feeds on a number of species of short grasses which are cut by a plucking motion of large lips. This means that shallow rooted grasses are selectively removed and at high population densities; overgrazing and soil erosion occurs.

Feeding time is about 5-6 hours in night and the rest of the time is spent in the water. They walk on the land for grazing. The animals (group size 10-15 to 150) share a common grazing range and return to water along the tracks during the night or early morning. The hippos feed almost exclusively on vegetation. The pigmy hippo is a browser (roots, grasses, shoots and fruits) in the tropical forests and the hippo is semi-aquatic grazer.

Nutrient requirements and feeding: The hippopotamus is non-ruminant pregastric fermenter and feed is digested in compartmented stomach but the process seems to be less efficient. The digestibility of fibre is intermediate in hippos between ruminants including camelid and hindgut fermenters. However, daily food requirement average 40 kg equal to dry weight of about 1-1.5 percent of body weight compared with 2.5 percent of other mammals. This is probably because the hippopotamus has ability to minimize its energy expenditure. The active feeding period is short and for the remaining time the hippo is resting or inactive in a supportive, stable warm medium. Even energy requirements for muscle tone are reduced. The hippo most often opens its mouth to yawn.

Feeding and Nutrition of Bears

Bears in zoos are natural clowns. They grow rapidly. Bears, though quadratic, possess ability to stand on their hindlimbs. They are trained to dance, ride bicycles and scooters and to do various gymnastics.

The ursids (family Ursidae and order Carnivora) as a group are remarkably adaptable. They are true omnivores and can maintain body condition and reproduction by relying on available feed sources. Because of this adaptation and the common practice of feeding a commercial omnivore preparation or dog food for captive ursids, a few nutritional problems have been reported.

Feeding Habits in Natural Habitat: Indian Sloth Bear

Indian sloth bear is an inhabitant of Eastern India, especially Assam. Feed of sloth bear in natural habitat includes fruits, roots, flowers, tubers, berries, insects of all sorts and honey. The chief diet consists of ber berries (*Zizyphus jujuba*), fruits of achar (*Buchanania latifolia*), various tendus or ebonies (Dyospyros), amaltas (*Cassia fistula*), jamun (*Eugenia jambolana*), figs (*Bengalensis glomerate*), bel (*Aegle marmelos*) and the flowers of mahua tree (*Bassia latifolia*), white ants, honey and insects of all sorts.

During the season, it is a common sight to see the bears competing with each other for mahua fleshy calyx and even get intoxicated as a result of eating flowers. They occasionally eat eggs where normal feed was deficient. Tame bears, even when quite young, will eat meat readily. In search of feed, bears constantly climb trees for fruits and to rob bees' nests. They knock comb on to the ground, descend and eat it there. They can climb any tree and not limited to those with rough bark.

In search of insects, they display great ingenuity. In attacking a white ants nest, they burrow into the base until core is reached, finer dust is dispelled by blowing, and the termites with considerable amount of earth are sucked into the mouth. Another method of getting insects and feed is carried out by turning stones in the bed of a *nala* and grub underneath with their blubberous lips.

Feeding and Nutrition of Rhinoceros

The name "rhinoceros" derives from distinctive horns on the snout. Unlike those of cattle, sheep and antelopes, rhino horns have no bony core and they are merely an aggregation of keratin fibres perched on roughened area on the skull. The Indian and Javan rhinos have only one horn on the end of the nose. Indian one-horned rhinoceros (*Rhinoceros unicornis*) is listed in Schedule I and Part I of the Wildlife (Protection) Act, 1972 with amendment in 2002.

Feeding behaviour: All rhinoceros are herbivores dependent on plant foliage and need a large amount of feed to support their bulky body. Because of their large size and hindgut fermentation, they can tolerate relatively high contents of fibre in their diet, but they prefer more nutritious leafy material (Mcdonald, 1984). Indian rhinos are mainly grazers, they use a prehensile upper lip to gather tall grasses and shrubs, but can fold the tip away when feeding on short grasses. Woody browse comprises about 20 per cent of their diet during winter period.

All rhinos are basically dependent upon water, drinking almost daily at small pools or rivers when these are readily available. Indian rhinos particularly spend long periods lying in water to have cooling effect.

Experimental feeding: Sixty day-feeding trial data suggests that when berseem is fed as roughage source, its amount should be restricted to avoid occurrence of obesity (Kumar et al., 2012).

Body weight of rhinoceroses 1636 – 1655 kg
Dry matter intake through concentrate mixture, 7 kg / day
Dry matter intake through wheat straw 4.85 to 5.54 kg / day
Dry matter intake through green fodder (three sources)
                    Sugarcane 6.72 kg / day or
                    Berseem 7.74 kg / day or
                    M.P.Chari 8.47 kg / day

Feeding and Nutrition of Blackbuck

Captive blackbucks (*Antelope cervicapra*) of 25-33 kg live weight were used in a feeding trial to know the level of concentrate supplementation needed for their optimum productivity. Fresh oat and berseem were offered *ad libitum* to all the blackbucks. Forage-only diet was inadequate in supply of energy, phosphorus and zinc. Supplementation of concentrates at the rate of 0.5% body weight was able to meet the requirement of these nutrients while 1.0% supplementation supplied excess energy and P. It was concluded that the feeding of concentrates to the captive blackbuck fed forage-based diets should be restricted to 0.5% of body weight (Das et al., 2013).

Feeding and Nutrition of Moles

Moles are a class of mammals belonging to the family Talpidae under the order Insectivora. The common mole (*Talpa europea*) is a small insectivore adapted to underground digging existence. The body size of moles vary according to locality and season; head and body together usually measuring about 14 cm besides tail of 3 - 3.5 cm. The body weight of different species ranges between 80 - 120 g, and, as is the case with most mammals, males are bigger than females. Moles have elongated skulls, small eyes, reduced tails and ears, and short fur, capable of lying forward or backward in keeping with their fossorial habits.

Feeds and feeding habits: Moles feed on soil invertebrates, which form 90% of their diet. Moles are active round the clock with 3 to 4 hourly rhythm of alternating rest and activity. Moles also feed on insects and insect larvae. Normal diet is earthworms. Approximately 20 percent of their feed is of plant origin which may include tulips, bulbus iris, carrots, parsnips, potatoes, peas, beans, vetch, oats, corn and wheat. Often such items form a substantial part of an individual's diet.

Feeding and Nutrition of Shrews

Shrews are small, mouse like mammal with short legs, a long pointed nose and long tail and form the biggest family in the order Insectivora. They weigh up to 35 g. The family also includes the world's smallest mammal (2 g).

General feeding habits: Shrews are insectivorous in their diet, but also behave as small time carnivores and eat a variety of invertebrate and even small vertebrate animals. The semi-aquatic species like Neomys and European water shrew also have access to crustaceans and other water creatures not normally available to ordinary shrews. In addition, many shrews also eat small quantities of seeds and other plant materials. Shrews are voracious feeders and soon starve if deprived of food. The saliva of some shrews has been found to contain toxic substances which enable them to kill large animals.

Feeding and Nutrition of Hedgehog

The hedgehog is an insect-eating mammal covered with spines. They have hollow hairs while porcupine (Small rat-like animal covered with spines that the animal can stick out if attacked) has sharp spines. When disturbed the hedgehog's hair turns stiff and the mammal rolls into a ball pulling the head inside as part of its defence mechanism from predators. It looks like a sea urchin. It feeds on insects, frogs, small snakes, eggs and chicken.

Indian pangolin (Scaly Anteater):   Food is ants and termites.

Otters are aquatic mammals and predators in the river. Presence of Otters is an indication of pollution-free water, healthy aquatic life and well guarded forests. Otters predate on fishes, crabs, oysters, lobsters, prawns and snakes. They are graded high on aquatic food chain. They are categorized under endangered species by the IUNC. Wildlife Protection Act of India 1972 had categorized Otters under Schedule II.

Care and feeding of offspring

Before going into the subject proper, let us know about maternal transfer of immunity to the offspring, importance of colostrum and compositional differences of milk of mammals.

Placental Classification

The placentas of eutherian mammals are classified according to two major characteristics: (1) placental shape and contact sites between fetal and maternal tissue, and (2) the number of cellular layers that separate maternal and fetal circulation systems. Classification of placenta is on the basis of histological (microscopic), structural organization and the layers between fetal and maternal circulation - 3 main groups: **(1) Haemochorial** - placenta where the chorion comes in direct contact with maternal blood, example, humans and rodents; **(2) Endotheliochorial** - maternal endometrial blood vessels are bare to their endothelium and these come in contact with the chorion, examples, dogs, cats, elephants; **(3) Epitheliochorial or synepitheliochorial**- maternal epithelium of the uterus comes in contact with the chorion, considered as primitive, examples, horses, pigs and ruminants.

Prenatal Passive Transfer of Maternal Immunity

Passive transfer of maternal antibodies to the fetus is determined by the structure of the fetomaternal barrier. The epitheliochorial placentas of species such as horses, swine and ruminants generally impede passage of antibodies from maternal to fetal circulation systems (Tizard, 2001). In these animals, passive transfer of antibodies is dependent on the ingestion and absorption of colostrum. The endotheliochorial placentation, which occurs in dogs and cats, has been estimated to allow 5-10% of maternal transplacental antibody transfer, while haemochorial placentation of humans and rodents allows significant transplacental antibody transfer.

   In contrast to other hind-gut fermenters such as equines, both Asian (*Elephas maximus*) and African (*Loxodonta Africana*) elephants have been found to develop endotheliochorial placentas. This architecture of placenta is associated with modest maternal to fetal transplacental antibody transfer. However, it remains unknown whether the bulk of passive immune transfer in elephants is achieved prenatally or postnatally through ingestion of colostrum. Zoo elephants are immunized with tetanus toxoid and /or rabies vaccine as part of their routine health care. Testing of serum samples collected from newborn Asian elephants at birth (before ingestion of colostrum), 2-4 days after birth and 2-3 months of age indicated that the newborn had anti-tetanus toxoid and anti-rabies titers that were equivalent to or higher than the titers of their dams (Nofs et al., 2013). The results demonstrated that the majority of passive transfer of maternal immunity occurs prenatally.

In mammals, maternal factors can be transferred via the placenta, in the colostrum and in normal milk during lactation. In birds, reptiles and fishes, maternal factors are mainly transferred via the egg to the offspring, hence the time period for the uptake of maternal factors is restricted to a period before, and shortly after birth. Maternal antibody transfer can have direct effects on offspring growth rate probably by passively protecting the newborn from common pathogens before their endogenous immune system has matured. Among the maternal factors that can be transferred by the mother to her offspring are hormones, antibodies and nutrients (macronutrients, mainly protein; micronutrients, e.g. carotenoids).

Parasites and other pathogens can have a decisive impact on the survival and performance of individuals hence protection against disease agents must be essential in natural populations. The humoral, antibody-mediated immune system matures slowly in neonatal vertebrates, restricting them to fighting off infections and parasites with the innate immune system. However, maternally transferred antibodies may constitute an important addition to the neonate's ability to take care of antigens. The vulnerable period in young vertebrates is from birth to the age when the youngster starts to synthesize antibodies endogenously. The age at which the neonate starts to produce antibodies on its own differs markedly between species (Grindstaff et al. 2003). In some birds, increases in the levels of antibodies have been found 10-14 days post-hatch, whereas it may take several weeks in poultry and rodents, and several months to years in humans.

The immune protection provided by maternally transferred antibodies is of rather short duration because they are catabolized. Most matAb may have disappeared from the offspring within 5-14 days in birds (Grindstaff et al. 2003, 2006), whereas in mammals lactation prolongs the period of passive protection to 5-10 weeks in rodents and approximately 9 months in humans. Hence, given that vertebrate neonates have a rudimentary immune defence early in life, the potential importance of matAb transfer to protect the neonate offspring from infection is considerable.

The evolutionary trend toward an increased reliance on prenatal antibody transfer in the higher primates appears to be most pronounced in the human infant, because our placenta has evolved an active transport process that elevates IgG in the full-term fetus over maternal levels. Higher IgG levels in the young infant ensure a more prolonged and successful period of passive immunity against pathogens previously encountered by the mother.

Colostrum is the Source of a Passive Immune System

The first milk produced during each lactation cycle is called colostrum. Because the neonate is borne into a very septic environment relative to the sterile uterus, development of an immune system is essential. Colostrum is often noted for its high concentration of maternal antibodies or immunoglobulins, active phagocytic cells, and bacteriocidal enzymes (Cockson and McNeice, 1980). The phagocytic cells and bacteriocidal enzymes are important to all neonates in countering infection of the gastrointestinal tract. However, the significance of colostral IgG immunoglobulins in providing circulating, passive immunity is species specific.

The secretion of colostral IgG immunoglobulins is practical only as long as the neonatal gut remains permeable to their absorption and upper-tract digestion of these proteins is minimal. The intestine of ungulates remains permeable to the intact immunoglobulin for only 24-36 hr after birth but continues in mink for 8 days, in mice and rats for 16-20 days, and in macropod marsupials for 170-200 days. The very prolonged absorption capability in marsupials corresponds to the time that the young reside in the pouch. Other types of immunoglobulins, such as IgA, continue to occur in milk after absorption of intact molecules has ceased and are important in protecting the neonatal gut from infection.

Milk Composition of Wild Mammals

The major constituents of milk are water, minerals, protein (such as casein), fat, and carbohydrates (Refer Table in the appendix). Protein concentration ranges from under 10 g/liter in some primates to over 100 g/liter in hares, rabbits, and some carnivores. Fat varies from traces in the milk of rhinoceroses and horses to over 500 g/liter in some seals and whales. Lactose, (a polymer of glucose and galactose) is the main carbohydrate of placental mammal milk. Lactose content ranges from traces in the milk of some marine mammals and marsupials to more than 100 g/liter in primates. Marsupial milk, nevertheless, can be very high in carbohydrates, but the sugars are primarily oligo- and poly-saccharides rich in galactose (Green, 1984).

Variation in milk composition: All these variations in milk composition between species reflect the compromises made to maximize the offspring's survival.

Aquatic mammals: The aquatic animals abstain entirely from eating or drinking during a relatively short but intense lactation. Most aquatic mammals produce highly concentrated milks. The reduction in milk water content in aquatic mammals provides a high-energy, low-bulk diet that is useful in offsetting neonatal heat loss in cold environments and conserves water in those mothers, such as the northern elephant seal. Seals that give birth on pack ice have very short lactation periods (e.g., hooded seals - 4 day lactation) or those that leave the neonate for feeding trips lasting several days produce more concentrated, higher-fat milks than do other seals.

Terrestrial mammals - Marsupials: For terrestrial mammals, the largest changes in milk composition over time occur in marsupials (Green, 1984). The embryonic marsupial confined to the pouch consumes dilute, high-sugar milk that, perhaps, provides nourishment similar to that occurring in the uterus of a eutherian during their longer gestation. Once the young begin leaving the pouch, the milk becomes more concentrated with more fat and protein and less sugar.

Eutherians: Most terrestrial eutherians produce milks that are intermediate in concentration to the nutrient-rich milk of aquatic mammals and the very dilute milks of primates (baboons, humans, lemus, talopoin monkey) and perissodactyls (ass, black rhinoceros, horse).

The milks of domestic cattle, goats, and camels contain about one-half the protein and energy per unit volume that occur in the milks of wild artiodactyls. These dilute milks from domestic artiodactyls are more similar to that produced by humans than they are to wild artiodactyls. Lactose, sodium and potassium are important regulators of the osmotic potential or water content of milk in the mammary gland. Hence, concentrated milks have either a low sugar (such as marine mammals) or mineral content while dilute milks have a higher sugar (such as primates and perissodactyls) or mineral content (Martin, 1984).

Composition of the milk fat and protein: The actual composition of the milk fat, protein, and sugar also differ between animals. For example, the fatty acids of most milk are dominated by palmitic (16:0) and oleic acids (18:1). However, the main fatty acid of lagomorphs (rabbit, hare) and elephant (proboscideans) milk is capric acid (10:0), which is synthesized in the mammary gland, whereas those of seal milk are long-chain unsaturated fatty acids (18:3 and higher) that are probably derived directly from the diet.

The amino acid taurine appears to be a dietary essential for most neonatal mammals, particularly carnivores. The taurine content of colostrum is usually higher than in mature milk. However, carnivores have much higher concentrations of taurine in the mature milk than do herbivores (cat -287 mol/100 ml; dog -181, domestic cow - 1, guinea pig - 17, rabbit - 14, sheep - 14, and horse 3). The sulfur containing amino acid content of tammar wallaby milk increases sharply coinciding the beginning of hair growth in the neonate. Casein composition or structure will determine the hardness of the milk clot formed in the stomach of the neonate and the rate at which nutrients are digested.

Peak Milk Production by Various Mammals

Milk production generally rises during early lactation to a peak before falling during the weaning process. Peak yields generally increase as a function of maternal metabolic body weight (exponents range from 0.67 to 0.81; Oftedal, 1984a). Litter-bearing species [American black bear (n=2.5) and guinea pigs (n=3.1)] with altricial young produce at least twice as much milk as do ungulates with a single offspring (Tammar wallaby and brown hare). Although bears and wallabies produce very altricial neonates, their developmental stage at the time of emergence from the pouch corresponds to that of a precocial neonate at birth.

Well-fed ungulates with twins generally produce 67% more milk than do those with a single offspring. The baboon and human produce the least milk, which corresponds with their very slow growth rates.

The decline in milk production once the peak has been reached can last for as little as 5 days in mice to many months in large ungulates.

Methods for determining milk intake: Weighing the neonate or the mother before and after a controlled nursing period and hand milking the lactating female and weighing the milk; using isotopes of hydrogen or sodium to quantify either the dilution of the neonate's body water or sodium pools by ingested milk or the actual transfer of these elements from the mother to the young via milk. Each method entails various assumptions or experimental and interpretational difficulties.

Nursing of the young: Some species - such as the tree shrew nourishes its young only once in 48 hr (Martin, 1966), while rabbits and hares suckle once in 24 hr (Linzell, 1972; Broekhuizen and Maaskamp, 1980).

Care and Feeding of Orphaned Neonates

Nutritionists working at zoos should be leaders in conducting well planned, scientifically based studies to understand the animals' basic biology. Studies of the mother-neonate interaction are essential to successfully raise orphaned wildlife.

Numerous attempts have been made to hand-raise orphaned wildlife. But the successful care of very young animals is still largely an art requiring dedication and perseverance. For example, many neonates do not defecate or urinate unless manually stimulated by rubbing or washing the anal and genital area. Faeces produced from the digestion of milk are normally quite soft and aromatic. Hence, their (faeces) consumption by the lactating female as she licks the infant ensures cleanliness when altricial infants are confined to a nest, den, or pouch (e.g. carnivores, rodents, or marsupials) and reduces the chance of attracting predators even to preococial neonates (e.g., artiodactyls).

Milk Formulation is one of the Major Concerns in Raising Orphans.

Lactose-intolerance: Excess or inappropriate milk sugars or fats can cause diarrhoea and digestive upsets. Lactose is a particular problem when using cow's milk or lactose-containing milk replacers to raise neonates of species, such as seals, in which the natural milk is largely devoid of this disaccharide. When lactose is fed to neonates in whom the enzyme lactase is inadequate for its digestion, severe diarrhoea occurs due to (1) bacterial growth and (2) the osmotic effect of undigested sugar in the intestine.

Use of galactose (a component of lactose) or lactose-containing formulas can also produce cataracts in neonates that do not normally encounter these sugars (e.g.seals). If cellular enzyme systems are inadequate to metabolise the absorbed galactose, this compound is converted to a sugar alcohol that is retained in the lens of the eye (Stephens, 1975).

Several milk substitutes that are lactose-free and galactose-free are available as a formula base for lactose-intolerant species. Many other deficiencies, particularly amino acids in very young mammals, and pathogens can cause cataracts (Vainisi et al., 1980). Disaccharide-intolerance and the debilitating consequences also can be produced by feeding other sugars. For example, sucrase, the enzyme necessary to digest common table sugar or corn syrup, is very low or absent in many mammalian neonates.

Added fats also produce severe diarrhoea: Added fats in the form of common cooking oils produce severe diarrhoea. If fat is to be added, butterfat is usually preferred. Other fats, such as animal tallow or egg yolk, can also be used. Coconut oil has been useful in developing formulas for young elephants as it more closely approximates the high concentration of medium-chain-length fatty acids in elephant milk than does butterfat that is dominated by long-chain fatty acids. Fats containing medium-chain-length fatty acids are more easily digested than fats containing long-chain fatty acids. If significant amounts of fat are added or if fat digestion is a problem, the milk fat may need to be emulsified or homogenized to reduce fat droplet size. Although elephant milk contains 2-3 times as much fat as does cow's milk, the fat droplets in elephant milk are one-half the size of those in raw cow's milk.

Formulation of Milk Replacer and Feeding

Although neonates have been successfully fed milk very dissimilar to the composition of the normal maternal milk, most neonates do better when fed milks similar to the normal milk. Milk replacers of any composition can be formulated because of availability of ingredients in pure form. While formulating milk replacers, the normal compositional changes that occur during lactation are to be kept in mind.

Once the best milk formula has been determined, the nutritionist must determine the amount to be fed, the method of feeding, and the feeding schedule. The amount fed should be based on a knowledge of neonatal milk intake control, requirements, and efficiencies of nutrient utilization. Many infants have been fed *ad libitum* quantities of milk with the assumption that the neonate would correctly control its intake. Milk is often ingested in excess of physiological capacities and results in diarrhoea, vomiting, listlessness, potbellies, laboured breathing, anorexia, and death.

Neonatal Milk Intake Control

Mother-raised Neonatal Ungulate Versus Bottle-Raised

Well-fed ungulate females during the first week of lactation often allow the offspring seemingly unlimited access to the udder, with the young terminating all nursing bouts by simply moving away voluntarily from the udder. Later, the mother increasingly rebukes advances and behaviourally terminates all nursing bouts by moving away or forcefully rejecting the young before it is willing to relinquish the teat. These observations suggest that the young ungulate is quite capable of controlling its own intake from the beginning, with the mother balancing her needs and resources with those of the neonate.

However, when the same neonatal ungulates are bottle-raised, they are incapable of correctly controlling their intake and, if initially given free access to milk, will drastically overeat and develop acute diarrhoea. The larger hole of most artificial nipples often delivers milk far faster than the maternal teat. Hence, it may not provide the time cues necessary for the neonate to sense or judge its state of fill.

Bottle-raised neonatals may encounter diarrhoea. It may be due to lack of knowledge about lactation and neonatal metabolism. Some of the diarrhoea is primarily pathogenic due to inadequate antibody transfer and totally independent of diet. But many have been found to be due to the use of improper milk replacers and feeding schedules that predispose the neonate to gastrointestinal infection. The prime need is correction of the dietary cause accompanied by treating diarhoea with antibiotics.

Milk intake control in young rats: Milk intake control between mother-raised and bottle-raised can be judged in light of milk intake control in young rats. The neonatal rat pup is often attached to the mother's teat for the majority of the day. However, attachment is not synonymous with milk intake and intake control. The 1-day-old pup is indeed incapable of correctly controlling its intake. Neonatal milk intake is controlled by the "continuous duet" between the pup and the mother, which only intermittently lets milk down into the nipple in response to the level of suckling stimulation provided by the pup (Epstein, 1986). The healthy pup will eagerly and almost reflexively consume all milk that the mother provides.

If the pup is given access to more milk during a sucking bout, such as by cannulating the mother's teat or pup's mouth and artificially providing more milk or inducing additional milk let-down in anesthetized mothers by prolonged, repeated oxytocin injections, milk is consumed until the physical capacity of the stomach forces milk into the intestinal tract as far as the large intestine. Similarly, milk will back up into the nose and mouth, and the pup will simply choke until it has cleared its respiratory tract of milk. Only the 15-to 20-day-old pup is able to control its intake correctly.

Need to understand the animal's basic biology before raising orphans: Mule deers versus mountain goats

Mule deer and mountain goats offer another example of the need to understand the animal's basic biology before raising orphans.

- Neonatal mule deer are "hiders" during their early life as they try to avoid predation by being very secretive. Mother does not stay with the fawn, but returns to the fawn from 2 to 10 times a day for nursing.

- Goats are "followers" as the mother provides an active defense against predation while nursing the neonate up to 40 times a day.

Fawns raised as singles by their mother consume between 150 and 200 g per nursing bout. Mountain goats, because of their more frequent nursing, consume only 50 g per feeding. The composition of the milk and the amount of milk consumed per day are similar for mule deer and mountain goats. However, bottle-raising protocols that use infrequent feedings (e.g., 4 per day) of large volumes (e.g., 150 ml per feeding) are very successful for mule deer but kill mountain goats. Feeding volumes larger than 90 ml will exceed the capacity of the goat's true stomach and may not be digested. Thus, mule deer fawns are anatomically and physiologically adapted for ingesting "meals" whereas goat kids have evolved to consume milk in "snack" proportions (Carl and Robbins, 1988).

14

Planning for Balanced Feeding - Wild Animals

Balanced Diet

A balanced diet is one which yields daily the nutrients in the proper amounts and proportions to satisfy the needs of the body under the various conditions. Cost of the diet has received adequate consideration. Thus least cost balanced diets have been arrived at by using linear programming, after using appropriate constraints consistent with practical consideration.

It should contain the various groups of foodstuffs such as energy yielding foods, body building foods and protective foods in the correct proportions so that the individual animal is assured of obtaining the minimum requirements of all the nutrients.

The components of a balanced diet will differ according to age, sex, physical activity, economic status and the physiological state, *viz* pregnancy, lactation etc.

Normally various food items are used in formulating nutritionally adequate diets for various categories of animals to meet their recommended allowances and also for formulating special diets for therapeutic purposes.

Feeding Zoo Animals

The challenge of a zoo nutrition programme is to provide a nutritionally balanced diet, which reasonably stimulates natural feeding behaviour and which is consistently palatable to the animals. Zoo nutrition must facilitate the captive animal management goals of reproduction, longevity, good health and behavioural normality (Das et al., 2012). Zoo nutritionist must ensure that the animals may get sufficient opportunity to choose their diet according to seasonal, physiological, environmental or individual needs. However, nutrient requirements of zoo / wild animals are very little known.

In most of the zoos, animals are fed empirically based upon whether they are herbivore, omnivore or carnivore. However, such a practice is not scientific considering the fact that many herbivores will gnaw and carnivores like panda will thrive on completely vegetarian diet (Das et al., 2012). Such empirical feeding practices followed in most of the zoos may either lead to under- or over-feeding which may ultimately result in various health hazards, reproductive disorders and reduced life-span.

Zoo animals in a group situation tend to be fed in excess of their requirements in order to ensure that the youngest or most subordinate animal obtains sufficient food, but some dominant animals may consume energy in excess of their requirement and become obese. In contrast, low level of food intake may occur in animals that experience severe seasonality in food intake in the wild. Even in captivity, the effect of photoperiod, temperature and other factors may induce period of chronic energy deficit and weight loss attributable to depressed intake (Ofteadal and Allen, 1997).

Fatty Acid Deficiency in Captive Animals

Freshly-harvested browses contained about 15 times higher concentrations of α-linolenic acid (an omega-3) than linoleic acid (an omega-6 FA). However, the fodder that is offered to captive animals showed to contain five-fold higher linoleic acid compared to α-linolenic acid. This imbalance in omega-3 and omega-6 fatty acids lead to deficiency and reflected in certain health disorders.

Mineral Deficiency in Captive Animals

Mineral imbalances have long been recognized in zoo species. The first documented nutritional problems in large carnivores fed meat-based diets, and primates and birds raised primarily on fruits were reported from the London Zoo. Many kinds of foods are low in calcium and have Ca: P ratio less than 1. Excessive use of fruits, seeds or grains and muscle meat (low calcium-high phosphorus foods) can have severe consequences for zoo animals. Demineralization of bone, tetany and eventual death may occur as animals deplete skeletal store of Ca. Grain and plant protein source contain more P than Ca, but much of the P may be unavailable as it is bound to phytate. Phosphorus deficiency may well be the most critical mineral deficiency in grazing mammals (Underwood and Suttle, 1999).

The apparent absorption coefficient for Ca ranges from 60-83% in case of rhino (Clauss et al., 2005) and 40-60% in elephants (Clauss et al., 2003).

Endogenous faecal Ca loss was calculated as 5.1 mg Ca/kg BW/day in rhino and 6.6 mg in elephant (Clauss, et al,. 2003). In such situation, absorption of a large proportion of Ca through GI tract, and excretion of the surplus via the kidney and urinary tract could overload with excess of Ca causing urolith (Das et al., 2012 textbook chapter).

The apparent absorption coefficient for phosphorus was between 12 and 29% in rhino and 10-30% in Asiatic elephant (Clauss et al., 2003). Endogenous P losses were 10 mg/kg BW for rhino and 6.0 mg/kg BW for Asiatic elephant.

A minimum of 0.7% Ca and 0.4% P is suggested for elk rations. Calcium to phosphorus ratio of at least 1.5 to 1 is needed. Hardened deer antlers contain about 22% calcium and 11% phosphorus. A diet of 0.64% Ca and 0.56% P is necessary for antler growth. Stags can store minerals in their skeletons, and transfer them to the antlers when needed. In fact, during antler mineralization, male deer undergo osteoporosis. The minerals lost from the bones are replaced from the diet after the antlers are hardened. Yearling hinds and stags have high nutritional demands for skeletal growth. Yearling stags have the added nutritional demand to grow their first set of antlers. Stags require high levels of Ca, P, trace minerals and protein for antler growth (Bass Pro, 2006-07).

Energy

Over-nutrition, with accompanying obesity, is a health issue for many captive psittacines, and may negatively impact reproduction in these species. Over-condition can also be problematic for health of zoo primates, carnivores, and herbivores leading to problems with diabetes, respiratory and cardiac distress, hypertension, hypercholesterolemia, foot/hoof problems, and reduced reproduction (Von Houwald and Flach, 1998).

Protein

Excess protein can prove detrimental to animal health. Within weeks of switching from a high (>40%) protein diet (DM) basis) to a low (<10%) protein nectar diet that better related to native diet composition, humming birds successfully reproduced (Brice and Grau, 1989). A wide variability exists in commercial nectar product composition, with protein ranging from 2 to >20% of DM and these ranges appear to encompass levels that can prove harmful to captive populations of nectarivores (Frederick et al., 2003).

Similarly, the vulturine parrot (*Psittrichas fulgidus*) experienced health problem associated with excessive dietary protein on diets containing approximately 20% crude protein (DM basis). Nitrogen balance trials confirmed that adults of this species can maintain protein balance on diets containing only 2% protein (Pryor et al., 2001). A similar trend regarding a link between diet and disease in the Goeldi's monkey, or callimico (*Callimico goeldii*) has also been observed. Diets containing more than 25% crude protein have been linked with kidney disease, poor growth and reproduction.

Diets for Zoo Animals

Diets for zoo animals were developed on the basis of food preferences of the free-ranging animals, domestic animal data and experience of the animal-keeper (Sanyal, 1892). Recently, Arora (2001) with the effort of Central Zoo Authority (CZA) compiled the feeding schedules of zoo mammals practiced in different zoos in the country. It is observed that the variation in feeding schedules among the different zoos is very high. It has become imperative to prepare a standard diet schedule for zoo animals that could be used by the zoos spread across the Indian Union.

Feeding Schedules of Carnivorous Mammals* (Scientific name and Schedule of the Wildlife Act are mentioned in parenthesis)

Name of the animal	Diet prescribed	Quantity per day	Additional supplements**
1. Indian Lion and Indian tiger (*Parnther leo persica*, *panther tigris*) (Schedule I Part I	Beef with bone	7 to 10 kg	Chicken 1 kg per week; 2 eggs weekly twice (Lion male and tiger male are given 2-4 kg beef extra)
	Liver	150 to 500 g	Tiger cub is given chicken and beef at 0.65 kg and 2.0 kg, respectively.
	Sri Venkateswara Zoological Park, Tirupati follow	Milk half litre and eggs 2nos are given in the morning	Beef without bone (and calcium supplement) of 4–8 kg (female) / 5–10 kg (male) is given in the afternoon.
2. Jaguar	Beef with bone and liver	4 kg and 150 g, respectively	---------
3. Leopard or panther	Beef without bone	3 to 4 kg	Chicken 1 kg per week

(*Panthera pardus*)	Liver	100 to 250 g	Leopard cub is given 1.5 kg beef/day
(Schedule I Part I)	Sri Venkateswara Zoological Park, Tirupati follow	Milk half litre and eggs 2nos are given in the morning	Beef without bone (and calcium supplement) of 3kg is given in the afternoon.
4. Wolf (*Canis lupus pallipes*) (Schedule I Part I)	Sri Venkateswara Zoological Park, Tirupati follow	Milk half litre and eggs 2nos are given in the morning	Beef without bone (and calcium supplement) of 2 kg is given in the afternoon.
5. Wild dog or dhole (*Cuon alpines*) (Schedule II, Part I)	Beef without bone Liver	2.5 kg 100 g	
(Hyena, wild dog)	Sri Venkateswara Zoological Park, Tirupati follow	Milk quarter litre and egg 1no are given in the morning	Beef without bone (and calcium supplement) of 2kg is given in the afternoon.
6. Hyena (*Hyaena hyaena*) (Schedule III)	Beef with bone Liver	3.0 kg 100 g	Chicken 500 g per week
7. Jackal (*Canis aureus*)	Beef without bone Liver	0.5 to 1.5 kg 100 g	Chicken 250g per week
(Schedule II, Part II)	Sri Venkateswara Zoological Park, Tirupati follow		Beef without bone (and calcium supplement) of 1kg and chicken liver 250 g are given in the afternoon.
8. Palm civet cat or toddy cat (Schedule II, Part II)	Beef with bone Or chicken Banana Milk Bread slices	100-300 g 2 nos/150 g 50 - 100 ml 2 nos/100 g	

Civet cat	Sri Venkateswara Zoological Park, Tirupati follow	Bread 20g, milk 200g and banana 100g are given in the morning.	Mutton 100g and egg 1no are given in the afternoon.

Aquatic mammal

9. Otter (*Luthra perspicillata*) (Schedule II, Part II)	Fish	1.5 kg	1.5 kg crab 300g weekly twice

10. Sloth bear	Ragi (cooked) Rice gruel with black gram	250 to 300 g 150 + 50 g to 300 g + 100 g, respectively	
(*Melursus ursinus*)	Orange/ mango fruits	2 nos	
(Schedule I, Part I)	Guava fruits	4 nos	
	Tapioca / sweet potato	100 g	
	Jaggery	250 g	
	Banana	5 Nos	
	Groundnut (w.o.s)	100 g	
	Honey	100 g	(Bi-weekly)
	Milk	500 ml	
	Bread slices	5 Nos	
	Carrot	200 g	
	Radish	100 g	
	Boiled egg	1 No	
	Cucumber	500 g	
	Tomato	250 g	
	Bengal gram	100 g	
	Seasonal fruits:		
	Water melon	500 g	
	Jackfruit	100 g	
	Sithaphal	100 g	
	Naval or Jamun	100 g	
	Sri Venkateswara Zoological Park, Tirupati follow	Banana 200g, sweetlime /orange 200g, guava/mango /pine apple 100g, papaya 100g, tomato 100g, bread 50g and honey 30g are given in the morning.	Sorghum and ragi mix (2:1) 1.5 kg, 100g black gram/green gram, milk 1 litre, carrot 250g, salt 50 g and egg 1no are given in the afternoon.

* Adapted from diet sheet during 2011-2012, Arignar Anna Zoological Park, Vandalur, Chennai-48; W.O.S= without shell; wild cats include tiger, lion, puma or cougar, jaguar, panther or leopard, lynx.

**Only iodised salt is provided for salt supplementation. Tuesday is fasting for all animals except pregnant animals, ailing animals, nursing animals and other special cases.

Feeding Schedules of Herbivorous Mammals* (Scientific name and Schedule of the Wildlife Act are mentioned in parenthesis)

Name of the animal	Diet prescribed	Quantity per day	Additional supplements**
Indian Elephants	Ragi cooked	20 kg	
(*Elephas*	Horse gram	4 kg	
maximus)	Rice	2kg	
(Schedule I,	Common salt	250 g	
Part I)	Joggery	250 g	
	Grass	200 kg	
	Sugarcane	12 nos	
	Green tree leaves-Bamboo	100 kg	
	Coconuts	4 Nos	
	Banana	10 Nos	
	Papaya	2 kg	
	Seasonal fruits:		
	Wood apple	500 g	
	Water melon	2 kg	
Elephant calves	Ragi cooked	6 kg	
	Horse gram	1 kg	
	Rice	1 kg	
	Joggery	250 g	
	Common salt	50 g	
	Banana	10 nos	
	Grass	75 kg	
	Sugarcane	4 nos	
	Green tree leaves - bamboo / stylo	25 kg	
	Coconuts	2 nos	
	Papaya	1 kg	
	Seasonal fruits:		
	Wood apple	250 g	
	Water melon	1 kg	

	Sri Venkateswara Zoological Park, Tirupati follow	Green grass 100kg, ragi, rice and horse gram balls (4:3:1) 4kg, common salt 75g, joggery 200g, tree fodder/coconut frond 50 kg and sugarcane 10kg as per the availability in the forenoon.	Green grass 100kg, ragi, rice and horse gram balls (4:3:1) 4kg, common salt 75g, joggery 200g, coconuts 2 nos, beetroots 2 kg and banana 3 kg in the afternoon.
Indian Porcupine#	Rice	100 g	
(Hystrix Indica) (Schedule IV)	Sri Venkateswara Zoological Park, Tirupati follow	Bengal gram 50g, potato 50g, carrot /beetroot 25g, banana 50g, cabbage 50 g, palak leaves 25 g and guava/mango /papaya 50g in the forenoon.	Bengal gram 50g, potato 50g, carrot/ beetroot 25g, banana 50g, cabbage 50 g, palak leaves 25 g and guava/mango/papaya 50g in the afternoon.
Indian Crested Porcupine; nocturnal animal	Carrot Cabbage Tapioca or sweet potato Soya chunks / soybeans Groundnut without shell Banana	100 g 100 g 100 g 20 g 50 g to 150 g 2 nos	
Hippopotamus	Wheat bran Bengal gram Common salt Apple Potato Carrot Cabbage Onion Banana Grass Greens Bread	10 kg 500 g 250 g 2 nos 500 g 2 kg 1 kg 250 g 10 nos 100 kg 1 kg 2 loaves (800g/ 40 slices)	

Pygmy hippo	Wheat bran	2.5 kg	
	Bengal gram	250 g	
	Common salt	50 g	
	Carrot	1 kg	
	Potato	250 g	
	Cabbage	250 g	
	Onion	100 g	
	Banana	5 nos	
	Apple	2 nos	
	Grass	10 kg	
	Greens	500 g	
	Bread slices	20 nos; 1loaf (400g)	
Indian gaur /Indian bison (Schedule I, Part I)	Wheat bran	3 kg	
	Cattle feed	3 kg	
	Horse gram boiled	750 g	
	Groundnut cake	1 kg	
	Banana	5 nos	
	White Bengal gram	500 g	
	Green gram sprouted	300 g	
	Common salt	100 g	
	Green grass	25 kg	
	Tree leaves	10 kg	
	Greens	500 g	
Giraffe	Sri Venkateswara Zoological Park, Tirupati follow	Sweet potato/ beetroot 4kg, carrot 2kg, onion 2 kg, beans 1kg, cowpea 500g, bengal gram 500g, banana 3kg, orange /sweet lime 2kg, guava/mango 500g and apple 1kg in the forenoon.	Giraffe mixture*** 5kg, common salt 30g, black salt 30g, joggery 200g and *ad lib* tree fodder (*Ficus bengalensis* leaves, jamun leaves, papal leaves etc; about 30kg) in the afternoon.
Blackbuck / Spotted deer or chital (*Axis axis*) Barking deer/	Wheat bran	0.5 kg to 1.5 kg	
	Cattle feed	0.5 kg to 1.5 kg	
	White bengal gram	25 g to 100 g	

Sambar deer (*Cervus unicolor*) (Schedule III)	Grass Green leaves Common salt Stylo /Lucerne Cabbage	7kg 3 kg 10 g 2 kg 100 g to 250 g	
Blackbuck (*Antilope cervicapra*) (Schedule I, Part I)	Sri Venkateswara Zoological Park, Tirupati follow	Banana 100g, palak leaves 100g, carrot /beetroot 500g, and *ad lib* green grass (about 3kg) in the forenoon.	Cattle feed 500g and *ad lib* green grass (about 3kg) in the afternoon.
Nilgai (*Boselaphus tragocamelus*) (Schedule III)	Wheat bran Cattle feed Bengal gram Green gram Groundnut cake Common salt Carrot Cabbage Greens Grass Green leaves	1.5 kg 1.5 kg 250 g 500 g 250 g 20 g 1 kg 250 g 500 g 20 kg 5 kg	
Nilgai, Sambar	Sri Venkateswara Zoological Park, Tirupati follow	*ad lib* green grass in the forenoon.	Cattle feed 1kg, carrot /beet root 0.5 kg and *ad lib* green grass in the afternoon.
Mouse deer (*Tragulus meminna*) (Schedule I, Part I)	Sri Venkateswara Zoological Park, Tirupati follow	Carrot 50g, banana 100g, apple 50g, sweet potato 50g, green leaves (palak) 100g and *ad lib* green grass are given in the forenoon.	Hay 0.5kg, sweet potato 50g, bengal gram 50g, green leaves (palak) 100g and *ad lib* green grass are given in the ofternoon.
Barking deer muntjac (*Muntiacus muntjak*) (Schedule III)	Sri Venkateswara Zoological Park, Tirupati follow	Cabbage 100g, green grass 3kg and palak/ amaranthus 250g are given in the forenoon.	Cattle feed 0.5kg, wheat bran 0.5kg, bengal gram 50g, groundnut cake 50g and common salt 10g in the afternoon.

Hog deer (*Axis porcinus*) (Schedule III)	Sri Venkateswara Zoological Park, Tirupati follow	Cabbage 100g, green grass 6kg and palak/ amaranthus 250g are given in the forenoon.	Cattle feed 0.5kg, wheat bran 0.5kg, bengal gram 100g, groundnut cake 100g and common salt 10g in the afternoon.
Swamp deer all sub-species *Cervus duvauceli*) (Schedule I, Part I)	Sri Venkateswara Zoological Park, Tirupati follow	Green grass 8kg and papal leaves *ad lib* are given in the forenoon.	Cattle feed 1.0kg, banana 200g and carrot /beetroot/sweet potato 500g are given in the afternoon.
Wild boar / wild pig (*Sus scrofa*) (Schedule III)	Wheat bran	500 g	
	Boiled rice	500 g	
	Bengal fram	100 g	
	Sweet potato / tapioca	200g	
	Bread slices	5 nos	
	Potato	250 g	
	Banana	5 nos	
	Common salt	10 g	
	Greens	100 g	
	Cabbage	250 g	
	Sri Venkateswara Zoological Park, Tirupati follow	Carrot 500g, sweet potato/pumpkin 500g, bengal gram /groundnut 200g, green leaves (palak /cabbage) 500g and green grass 1 kg are given in the forenoon.	Sorghum and ragi gruel 1.5kg and common salt 10g are given in the forenoon.

* Adapted from diet sheet during 2011-2012, Arignar Anna Zoological Park, Vandalur, Chennai-48. # Porcupine is a small rat-like animal covered with spines that the animal can stick out if attacked.

**Only iodised salt is provided for salt supplementation. Tuesday is fasting for all animals except elephants, pregnant animals, ailing animals, nursing animals and other special cases.

*** Giraffe mixture consists of cattle feed 2 kg, wheat bran 1 kg, maize 1kg, oats 0.5 kg and sunflower cake 0.5 kg.

Feeding Schedules of Primates* (Scientific name and Schedule of the Wildlife Act are mentioned in parenthesis)

Name of the animal	Diet prescribed	Quantity per day	Additional supplements**
Bonnet macaque (*Macaca radiata*) (Schedule II, Part I)	Rice	50 g	
	Groundnut wos	15 g	
	Banana	3 nos	
	Orange / mango	100-150 g	
	Guava	100 g	
	Bengal gram	15 g	
	Cabbage	50 g	
	Greens	100 g	
	Boiled egg	1 no on alternate days	
	Soya chunks	20 g	
	Carrot	25 g	
	Grapes	50 g	
	Honey	10 g	
	Seasonal fruits	25 to 50 g each	Sitapal, watermelon, jack fruit, *naval, nelli,* etc
Bonnet macaque /rhesus macaque (*Macaca mulatta*)/ stump-tailed macaque (*Macaca speciosa*) (Schedule II, Part I)	Sri Venkateswara Zoological Park, Tirupati follow	Egg 1no, Bengal gram 75g, carrot 50g, cabbage 50g, banana 200g, sweetlime 100g, guava/mango/pine apple 140g, papaya 200g, palak leaves 100g, bread 50g and groundnut 50g are given in the morning.	Banana 200g and guava etc fruits 70g are given in the afternoon.
Common langur (*Presbytis entellus*) (Schedule II, Part I) Nilgiri langur (*Presbytis johni*) (Schedule I,	Rice	30 g	
	Groundnut wos	25 g	
	Banana	4 nos	
	Orange / mango	1 no	
	Guava	1 no	
	Bengal gram	15 g	
	Cabbage	30 g	
	Greens	100 g	

Part I)	Bread slices	4 nos	
	Boiled egg	1 no (alternate days)	
	Soya chunks	20 g	
	Carrot	25 g	
	Grapes	20 g	
	Honey	10 g	
	Seasonal fruits	25 to 50 g each	Sitapal, watermelon, jack fruit, *naval, nelli,* etc
Common langur	Sri Venkateswara Zoological Park, Tirupati follow	Egg 1no, carrot 50g, cabbage 50g, banana 200g, sweetlime 100g, guava/mango/pine apple/papaya 140g, palak leaves 100g, and groundnut 50g are given in the morning.	Bread 50g, Bengal gram 75g, banana 200g and guava etc fruits 70g are given in the afternoon.
Olive baboon	Sri Venkateswara Zoological Park, Tirupati follow	Egg 1no, carrot 50g, cabbage 25g, Bengal gram 100g, banana 200g, sweetlime 100g, guava/mango/pine apple/papaya 140g, palak leaves 50g, and groundnut 50g are given in the morning.	Bread 50g, banana 200g and guava etc fruits 70g are given in the afternoon.
	Nocturnal primate		
Slender lories	Banana	2 nos	
	Bread slices	2 nos	
	Boiled egg	1 no	
	Grapes	125 g	
	Milk	100 ml	

| | Sri Venkateswara Zoological Park, Tirupati follow | Egg 1no and a few insects are given in the morning. | Apple 50g, banana 200g, bread 2 slices and minced meat 100g are given in the afternoon. |

* Adapted from diet sheet during 2011-2012, Arignar Anna Zoological Park, Vandalur, Chennai-48.

** Only iodised salt is provided for salt supplementation. Tuesday is fasting for all animals except pregnant animals, ailing animals, nursing animals and other special cases.

Feeding Schedules of Reptiles* (Scientific name and Schedule of the Wildlife Act are mentioned in parenthesis)

Name	Diet prescribed	Quantity per day	Additional supplements**
Marsh crocodile (*Crocodilus porosus*)	Fish, weekly once to twice	250 g	
	Beef with bone	500 g weekly once	
Salt water crocodile (*Crocodilus palustris*)	Fish weekly once	1 kg	
	Beef with bone	4 kg weekly twice	
(Schedule I Part II)	Sri Venkateswara Zoological Park, Tirupati follow	Dead fish 250g is offered in the forenoon.	Beef without bone 500g is given in the afternoon.
American alligator	Fish (weekly once)	1 kg	
	Beef with bone	3 kg weekly twice	
Python (Genus pybhon) (Schedule I, Part II)	Chicken	1 kg (twice in a month)	
	Or rat 150g size	8 nos (twice in a month)	
	Sri Venkateswara Zoological Park, Tirupati follow	Live bird of 500g is offered once a week in the forenoon	

Python sub-adult	Chicken	Half a kg (twice in a month)	
	Or rat 150g size	4 nos (twice in a month)	
Indian cobra (all sub-species of the genus Naja) (Schedule II, Part II)	Chicks	3 nos (weekly once)	
	Or rats 100 to 150 g	4 nos (weekly once)	
Common monitor lizard (*Varanus flavescens*) (Schedule I, Part II)	Rats	1 no (weekly once)	
	Or Chick & Chopped beef	2 nos (weekly once) 100 g (except Tuesdays)	
Iguana	Carrot	50 g	
	Cabbage	50 g	
	Tomato	50 g	
	Greens	100 g	
Star tortoise	Carrot	30 g	
	Cabbage	30 g	
	Tomato	30 g	
	Greens	50 g	
	Sri Venkateswara Zoological Park, Tirupati follow	Carrot 5g, bengal gram 5g, palak leaves 5g, papaya 5g are given in the forenoon	Carrot 5g, bengal gram 5g, palak leaves 5g, papaya 5g are given in the afternoon

* Adapted from diet sheet during 2011-2012, Arignar Anna Zoological Park, Vandalur, Chennai-48.

**Only iodised salt is provided for salt supplementation. Tuesday is fasting for all animals except pregnant animals, ailing animals, nursing animals and other special cases.

Feeding of sick animals (see also chapter 5 in cat and dog nutrition)

- Most seriously ill wild animals refuse to eat or just pick at the food. Force feeding often may not be practicable especially in carnivores or herbivores.

- Soft diet like chicken preferably in cooked form may be attempted as one of the significant diets in wild animal species.
- Intravenous fluids like dextrose saline, ringers lactate, etc. may be chosen in wild animals that have totally stopped eating activities.
- Attempts may be done to provide the most palatable food for the targeted wild animal species.
- In wild animals especially carnivores with severe gastritis whatever food is offered or ingested, it may be vomited often. In such cases, bland diet may be offered. Egg white may be offered to carnivores with severe vomiting, in addition to administration of 5% dextrose saline solution.
- Provision of bland diet in small quantities several times may help to minimize the incidences of vomiting or rejection by the concerned wild animal species.
- Provide drinking water *ad libitum* to all the sick wild animals in general.

Geriatric animal feeding (see also chapter 4 in cat and dog nutrition)

- Avoid feeding with less digestible feeds.
- Avoid full stomach feeding.
- Provide adequate quantities of vitamins and minerals.
- Provide water *ad libitum*.

Table 1. Chemical Composition of Common Foodstuffs (All values are per 100 g of edible Portion)*

Name of the foodstuff	1 Moisture g	2 Protein g	3 Fat g	4 Fibre g	5 Energy kcal	6 Ca mg	7 P mg	8 Fe mg
1. Cereals (Bajra, sorghum, Maize, Ragi, Rice, Wheat)								
	13.2	9.8	2.3	1.8	345	79	269	4.0
* exclusive of Ragi						26*		
2. Dhals (Bengalgram, blackgram, green gram, redgram)								
	11.8	22.9	2.5	1.1	351	90	356	3.9
3. Peas dry	16.0	19.7	1.1	4.5	315	75	298	7.1
4. Rajmah	12.0	22.9	1.3	(4.8)	346	260	410	5.1
5. Soybean	8.1	43.2	19.5	3.7	432	240	690	10.4
6. GLV: Amaranth group (Amaranth, Coriander, Fenugreek, Mint)								
	84.5	4.3	0.7	1.5	50	275	64	9.2
7. Agathi group (Agathi, drumstick, Ponnaganti)								
	75.5	6.7	1.3	2.0	86	690	70	2.1

8. Cabbage	91.9	1.8	0.1	1.0	27	39	44	0.8
Root & tubers								
9. Potato	74.7	1.6	0.1	0.4	97	10	40	0.5
10. Onion	86.6	1.2	0.1	0.6	50	47	50	0.6
11. Carrot	86.0	0.9	0.2	1.2	48	80	530	1.0
12. Radish white	94.4	0.7	0.1	0.8	17	35	22	0.4
Other vegetables								
13. Brinjal	92.7	1.4	0.3	1.3	24	18	47	0.4
14. Beans	82.0	4.7	0.4	2.8	49	113	81	1.7
15. Drumstick	86.9	2.5	0.1	4.8	26	30	110	0.2
16. Ladies finger	89.0	1.9	0.2	1.21	35	66	56	0.35
17. Plantain green	83.2	1.4	0.2	0.7	64	10	29	6.3
18. Plantain stem	88.3	0.5	0.1	0.8	42	10	10	0.1
19. Gourds (bitter gourd, bottle gourd, ridge gourd, snake gourd)								
	95.0	0.7	1.8	0.7	18	22	32	0.7
20. Groundnut kernel	3.0	25.3	40.1	3.1	567	90	350	2.5
21. Gingelly seeds	5.3	18.3	43.3	2.9	563	1450	570	9.3
22. Banana, ripe	70.1	1.2	0.3	0.4	116	17	36	0.4
23. Grapes	79.2	0.5	0.3	2.9	71	20	30	0.5
24. Guava	81.7	0.9	0.3	5.2	51	10	28	0.3
25. Tomato, ripe	94.0	0.9	0.2	0.8	20	48	20	0.6
26. Fish (Seer)	72.7	22.5	4.0	–	126	71	572	5.4
27. Egg	73.7	11.3	10.2	–	143	60	220	2.1
28. Mutton, muscle	71.5	18.5	13.3	–	194	150	150	2.5
29. Milk	87.5	3.2	4.1	–	67	120	90	0.2
30. Jaggery	3.9	0.4	0.1	–	383	80	40	2.6

* Adapted from "Nutritive Value of Indian Foods" 1989, NIN, Hyderabad.

Table 2. **Energy and protein content of common foodstuffs (per 100 g of edible portion)***

Foodstuff	Energy (kcal)	Protein (g)
Rice, raw, milled	345	6.8
Wheat, whole	346	11.8
Cereals, average	345	9.8
Bengalgram dhal	372	20.8
Blackgram dhal	347	24.0
Greengram dhal	348	24.5
Redgram dhal	335	22.3
Peas, dry	315	19.7
Rajmah	346	22.9
Soybean	432	43.2

Green leafy vegetables
   Amaranth group (Amaranth, Coriander, Fenugreek, Mint)

	50	4.3
Drumstick group (Drumstick leaves, Agathi, Ponnaganti)		
	86	6.7
Cabbage	27	1.8
Roots & tubers		
Potato	97	1.6
Onion	50	1.2
Carrot	48	0.9
Radish	17	0.7
Other vegetables		
Beans (average)	49	4.7
Brinjal	24	1.4
Ladies finger	35	1.9
Drumstick	26	2.5
Plantain green	64	1.2
Plantain stem	42	0.5
Average for gourds	18	0.7
Nuts & oilseeds		
Cashewnut	596	21.2
Groundnut	567	25.3
Coconut, fresh	444	4.5
Gingelly seeds	563	18.3
Mustard seeds	541	20.0
Fruits		
Apple	59	0.2
Banana	116	1.2
Grapes	71	0.5
Orange	48	0.7
Papaya	32	0.6
Tomato, ripe	20	0.9
Guava	51	0.9
Lemon	57	1.0
Egg	143	11.3
Fish(Seer)	126	22.5
Mutton, muscle	194	18.5
Milk (4.1% fat)	67	3.2
Curd	60	3.1
Cheese (40.3% moisture)	348	24.1
Butter (19% moisture)	729	–
Sugar	400	0.1
Jaggery	383	0.4

Chillies, green	29	2.9
Chillies, dry	246	15.9
Coriander	288	14.1
Fenugreek seeds	333	26.2
Garlic, dry	145	6.3
Pepper, dry	304	11.5
Tamarind pulp	283	3.1
Turmeric	349	6.3

* Adapted from "Nutritive value of Indian Foods "1989, NIN, Hyderabad

Table 3. Indian foods rich in calcium

Foodstuff	mg/100g
Ragi grain	344
Amaranth seeds	510
Bengalgram whole	202
Horsegram whole	287
Rajmah, Soybean	260
Gingelly seeds	1450
Mustard seeds	490
Agathi GLV	1130
Amaranth GLV	397
Fenugreek GLV	395
Cow Milk	120
Buffalo Milk	210
Cheese	790
Khoa	956

The oxalic acid present in certain foodstuffs (Table 4) form insoluble calcium salt making it unavailable for absorption.

Table 4. Some foodstuffs (oxalic acid content-wise in descending order)

Foodstuff	Content, mg/100g
Gingelly seeds	1700
Amaranth (tender) GLV	772
Plantain green vegetable	480
Horsegram grain	417
Almond, cashewnut	300–400
Amla fruit	296
Tamarind leaves, tender	196
Gogu, curry leaves, Drumstick leaves, Drumstick vegetable	101

Beet root	40
Seethaphal, mango fruits	30
Bajra grain	21
Potato	20
Tomato ripe	4
Tomato green	2
Cow milk	2

Table 5. Some foodstuffs (phytin phosphorus-wise in descending order)

Maize grain	85 % of P as Phytin P
Wheat grain and wheat flour	80 % of P as Phytin P
Coriander seed	81 % of P as Phytin P
Sorghum grain	77 % of P as Phytin P
Ragi grain	74 % of P as Phytin P
Curry leaves and drumstick leaves	60 % of P as Phytin P
Rice, bajra, all pulses and legumes, guava fruit	40-50 % of P as Phytin P
Fenugreek seeds, pepper, drumstick vegetable, plantain green	30-40 % of P as Phytin P
Potato, papaya ripe, pomegranate, banana ripe, chilies dry and rohu fish	10 % of P as Phytin P

Table 6. Total and beta-carotene contents of some foodstuffs*

Sl. No.	Name of the Foodstuff	Total carotene	Beta-carotene
1.	Agathi	45,000	15,440
2.	Amaranthus gangeticus, tender	20,160	8,340
3.	Drumstick leaves	42,000	19,690
4.	Carrot	8,840	6,460
5.	Sweet Potato (Yellow)	2,200	1,810
6.	Guava, country	400	0
7.	Mango, ripe	2,210	1,990
8.	Orange	2,240	190
9.	Tomato, ripe	3,010	590

* All values are µg per 100 g of edible portion, based on HPLC analysis.

Table 7. The chemical composition (%) of different milks

Nutrients	Human	Cow	Buffalo	Goat
Proteins, g	1.2	3.3	3.8	3.3
Fat, g	3.8	3.7	7.5	4.1
Lactose, g	7.0	4.8	4.4	4.7
Calories, kcal	7.1	69	100	76
Ash, g	0.21	0.72	0.8	0.77
Calcium, mg	33	125	210	130
Phosphorus, mg	15	96	130	106
Iron, mg	0.15	0.10	0.2	0.05
Vitamin A, ug	48	47	60	36
Thiamin, mg	0.02	0.04	0.05	0.05
Riboflavin, mg	0.04	0.18	0.10	0.12
Nicotinic acid, mg	0.17	0.08	0.28	0.20
Folic acid, ug	1.3	5.6	3.3	0.7
Vitamin B_{12}, ug	0.03	0.5	0.3	0.1
Ascorbic acid, mg	4.0	2.0	2.5	2.0

15

Effect of Processing on Nutritive Value of Foodstuffs

I Cooking

Wet Method and Dry Method

We eat most of the foods only after cooking except some vegetables (carrot, radish, etc.) and fruits. Cooking is of two types: wet method and dry method. Wet methods of cooking are boiling, steaming or pressure cooking. Pressure cooking reduces the cooking period and destruction of nutrients is minimum in the process. Dry methods of cooking are frying, roasting and baking and these are done at high temperature.

Cooking has both adverse and beneficial effects. The loss of nutrients on cooking depends on the temperature, duration of cooking and the nutrient. Cooking process differ not only from region to region but also from house to house. In a mixed diet, we obtain vitamins and minerals essentially from vegetables, and these nutrients are lost to varying degrees depending on how they are cooked.

When foodstuffs like cereals, pulses, flesh foods etcetera are boiled in plain water, there is no possibility of the loss of carbohydrates, proteins and fats. Some proteins may be lost if salt water is used for boiling vegetables and the cooking water is discarded. Similarly some of the mineral salts and vitamins that are soluble in water would be lost if the cooked water is thrown away. Sodium, potassium and calcium are commonly lost due to leaching. More than the minerals, it is the vitamins especially those of water soluble 'B' group which show a greater loss during cooking. Cooking in acid media with tamarind and other acids has a protective effect against vitamins.

Vitamin A and carotene are not lost during wet cooking. When foods are fried in oil, there can be a loss of vitamin A to the extent of nearly 75%. Leafy vegetables contain plenty of `carotene' which is converted to vitamin A in the body. Therefore it would be better if leafy vegetables are boiled in water than fried. They can be cooked by boiling in just enough water and seasoned.

When chips are fried, not much loss of vitamin A occurs because generally they are fried in oil for a very short time.

Sometimes baking soda is added to facilitate cooking of pulses. This practice leads to loss of some B-vitamins.

In case of root vegetables (e.g. potatoes), cooking them with skin prevents leaching of nutrients.

Vitamin C is lost during exposure of cut vegetables.

Eggs appear to suffer little loss in nutritive value during conventional cooking.

If fat is repeatedly heated during frying, it may contain toxic substances due to peroxidation and rancidity. Excessive heating may lead to browning/maillard reaction affecting the availability of amino acids.

Beneficial Effects of Cooking

1. It improves the appearance and palatability of foods and confers new flavours.
2. Cooking destroys harmful food-borne microorganisms. It destroys avidin (Present in raw egg white), trypsin inhibitor of duck eggs (Present in its white portion) and trypsin inhibitor and other antinutritional factors of certain feeds. Thus it improves the nutritive value of foods.
3. Stewing improves the absorption of vitamins: A general belief that raw or lightly cooked vegetables provide more vitamins for the body has been disproved now, at least for carotenoids. Boiling softens plant cells and improve the gut's absorption of carotenoids, the antioxidants which combat tissue damage and narrowing of the arteries.

Carotenoids	Source
Beta carotene	Carrot, broccoli, spinach
Lutein	Yellow and green vegetables
Lycopene	Tomatoes, water melons

The body is able to absorb 3 to 4 % of the carotenoids in raw carrots but the absorption increases fivefold if they are cooked and mashed. Thus cooking has several advantages in improving the quality, digestibility and palatability. At the same time, cooking also can reduce the vitamin and mineral content, but taking certain precautionary measures like cooking in limited water and in the presence of acids, it can help preserve vitamins to a great extent.

How to Prevent Loss of Nutrients Due to Cooking?

- Food should be cooked for as short a period as possible.
- It is advisable either to cook vegetables in a minimum amount of water or to use the cooking water in soups and gravies.
- It is recommended that the root vegetables are cooked with their skin and peel them before using them in other preparations if needed.
- It is advisable to cut vegetables into larger pieces and put them into boiling water immediately and cook for a short period in a vessel covered with a lid and to consume as soon as possible.
- It is a desirable practice to use a minimum quantity of fat for frying and avoid using it over and over again.

Washing with cold water removes B-vitamins (B_1 and niacin mainly) present in raw-milled rice to an extent of about 80% but only to 30% in case of parboiled-milled rice. Hence it is a good practice to wash with minimum amount of water and cooking it in sufficient amount of water so that all the water is absorbed and no 'ganjee' is discarded. The losses are less in parboiled-rice because during parboiling the nutrients diffuse into the grain and protective gelatinized starch coating is formed on the grain preventing leaching.

II Parboiling of Rice

Parboiling is a hydrothermal treatment followed by drying before milling for the production of milled parboiled grain. Dehusking of parboiled rice is easy and the grain becomes tougher resulting in reduced losses during milling. The most important change during parboiling is the gelatinisation of starch and disintegration of protein bodies in the endosperm. The starch and protein expand and fill the internal air space. The fissures and cracks in the endosperm are sealed, making the grain translucent and hard as a result of which the breakage of grain during milling is minimized to 10%.

The vitamin content is increased. Water dissolves the vitamins and minerals present in the hull, and the bran coat carries them into the endosperm. So loss of B_1, B_2 and niacin due to milling and polishing is comparatively low in the parboiled-rice than raw-rice. Parboiled-rice bran has higher oil content compared to raw-rice bran.

III Extrusion Technology

It has a significant role to play in developing countries to make cheap 'Ready-to-Eat (RTE) foods, based on inexpensive feed materials like broken rice, tubers, oilseed extract (an inexpensive source of starch, protein and fat) fortified with vitamins and minerals.

The extruders are devices to cook by mechanical means (Shear-cooking), which is highly energy efficient. The heat generated by shear effectively gelatinizes the starch, denatures the proteins and make 'carbohydrate-lipid complex' and 'protein-lipid complex' for taste and mouth - feel. Extrusion technology effectively utilizes the hidden - fat in cereals to form these complexes, without the need of added fat. The product is pasteurized, as no microorganisms can survive high temperature short residence time (HTST) effect in the barrel of extruder. Moreover, anti- nutritional factors like trypsin inhibitors, bitter principles, etc. are destroyed during extrusion. The extruded product is amenable to packaging and has a long shelf life due to destruction of lipase and other fat - splitting enzymes during extrusion. The retention of natural antioxidants like tocopherols and lecithins (in oilseed extracts) also prevents the rancidity. The extruded product after pulverizing may be used as drinks or porridges. These are ideal products in disaster relief, school - feeding and nutritional supplementation/intervention programmes.

16

Hygienic Preparation, Preservation and Storage of Foods

Important Causes for Food Becoming Unsafe

We must give due attention to the nutritive value of feed as well as to food hygiene for maintaining good health of the animals. There can be 3 important causes for food becoming unsafe: (1) Lack of care with regard to selection of food ingredients and their storage, (2) poor personal hygiene and (3) dirty surroundings. Buy only good foodstuffs fit for consumption. Vegetables and fruits should be washed well before cooking/eating. Foodstuffs brought home must be stored properly. Dry ventilated places are best for storage of perishables. Exposure to moisture can result in degeneration and fungus may develop on foodstuffs.

Hygienic Preparation

In order to protect the health of the consumer, the Government of India promulgated the 'Prevention of Food Adulteration Act' (P.F.A. Act) in 1954. The act prohibits the manufacture, sale and distribution of not only adulterated foods but also foods contaminated with toxicants and misbranded foods.

Standards for ensuring quality of products: Apart from the PFA Act (1954) and Fruit Products Amendment Order (1961), 'Agmark' Standards and Bureau of Indian Standard (BIS) specifications ensure that good quality products are marketed.

Food Adulteration

Foodstuffs		Common adulterants
1. Cereals -	Wheat, rice etc.	Stones and mud
	Wheat flour	Tapioca flour
2. Pulses		
	Bengal gram dhal	Khesari dhal (*Lathyrus sativus*)
	Red gram dhal	Khesari dhal coloured yellow with coaltar dye
	Bengal gram flour	Tapioca flour or starch coloured yellow with dye
3. Turmeric powder		Lead chromate powder
4. Chilli powder		Saw dust, brick powder
5. Mustard seeds		Argemone seeds
6. Black pepper		Dried papaya seeds
7. Coffee powder		Used coffee powder, roasted husk or date seed or tamarind seed powder
8. Vanaspati		Animal fat and other high melting fats
9. Vegetable oils		Argemone oil, mineral oil, cheap non-edible oils

Argemone poisoning: Use of edible oil adulterated with argemone oil lead to swelling of the body (dropsy) and rash, and death in some cases due to heart failure.

Lead chromate mixed with turmeric powder could result in stiffness of limbs due to lead poisoning.

Coaltar dyes and non-permitted colours in dhals or sweets may finally lead to cancer.

Mineral oils used as adulterants in edible oils could also cause cancer.

Contamination of Foods with Toxic Chemicals, Pesticides and Insecticides

1. Accidental mixing of the food with toxic chemical used as rat poisons such as arsenic oxides, barium carbonate, lead arsenate and others.
2. Accidental contamination with pesticides and insecticides.
3. The presence of some toxic chemicals or minerals in certain marine foods (eg. mercury).
4. Presence of excessive amounts of certain food additives such as metabisulphite, benzoic acid and sorbic acid in processed foods.
5. Presence of residues of animal feed additives such as diethyl stilbesterol and antibiotics in meat, milk of animals.

Contamination of Foods with Harmful Microorganisms

Raw foods such as meat, fish, milk, vegetables grown on sewage and purchased from the market are likely to be contaminated with harmful microorganisms such as bacteria (Clostridia, Salmonella, Shigella, Staphylococci, Streptococci), fungi (*Aspergillus flavus, Claviceps purpuria,* Fusarium and Penicillium) and parasitic (*Trichinella spiralis, Ascaris lumbricoides, Entamoeba histolytica, Ancylostoma duodenale*). These are generally destroyed during cooking or processing of food. Some of the microorganisms may survive due to inadequate heat processing. Improper storage of foods also attracts growth of microbes which can cause serious illness.

Spoilage of Foods

Foods are classified into three groups on the basis of ease of spoilage.

1. Stable or non perishable foods
   e.g., sugar, grains, dry products
2. Semiperishable foods
   e.g., potatoes, onions, fruits and vegetables having thick skin.
3. Perishable foods.
   e.g., meat, fish, milk, eggs and most fruits and vegetables.

The spoilage of foods may be caused by moulds, yeast, bacteria, enzymes, food constituents and insects.

Moulds: Some of the common moulds are Aspergillus, Penicillium, Rhizophus and Helminthosporium.

Yeasts are very useful in making bread, beer, wine, vinegar and many other fermented products. They are undesirable when they grow on fruits, fruit juices, squashes etc. Yeasts thrive best in light sugar solutions. During active fermentation yeast can be easily recognised by the formation of bubbles or foam at the surface of the product. Boiling destroys yeast cells and spores effectively. e.g., Saccharomyces, Candida etc

Method of Preservation

1. **Asepsis:** Packaging of food is a widely used application of asepsis.
2. **Filtration & pressure:** By this microorganisms are removed. The liquid is filtered through a previously sterilized "bacterial proof" filters using positive or negative pressure. This method has been used successfully with fruit juices, beer, soft drinks and water. Similarly,

washing or trimming of fruits and vegetables prior to processing reduces the load of microorganisms.

3. **Fermentation:** Decomposition of carbohydrates by microorganisms or enzymes is called fermentation. By this method, the foods are preserved by the organic acid formed by microbial action. Vinegar is used to preserve certain foods.

4. **Heat processing:** It is applied to solid canned packs of fruits and vegetables. (a) Pasteurization and (b) Heat at about 100°C or above 100°C

5. **Refrigeration:** Low temperatures are used to retard chemical reactions, action of food enzymes and to slow down or stop growth and activity of microorganisms in food.

6. **Drying:** Sun drying of foods.

7. **Preservatives:** "Preservative" means a substance which when added to food, is capable of inhibiting, retarding or arresting the process of fermentation, acidification or other decomposition. Several preservatives are used in preservation of syrups, jams, jellies, pickles, sauces etc.

   (i) **Sugar:** Sugar acts as a preservative in syrups, jams and jellies at a concentration of 65% or above by action of osmosis.

   (ii) **Salt:** Salt acts by osmosis. 10-15% conc. is sufficient to preserve most products. It inhibits enzymatic browning, discolouration and acts as an antioxidant too. It is also used for curing of fish & pork. Salt in the form of brine is used for canning, and pickling of vegetables.

   (iii) **Vinegar or acetic acid:** It checks aerobic and anaerobic fermentation. It possesses germicidal and antiseptic properties. It is used in the preservation of pickles, sauces, chutnies, meat, fish etc. It is also a useful tool to modify taste and flavour. The dose is 2%.

   (iv) **Benzoic acid and its salts:** Benzoic acid is sparingly soluble in water. Hence sodium benzoate is used. It preserves most fruit products (pH 3.5-4.0) at 0.06-0.10% concentration. Soft drinks are preserved with 600 ppm of benzoic acid and 350 ppm of SO_2. In the long run, the benzoate may darken the products.

   (v) **Sulphurous acid and its salts:** It is mostly administered in the form of its salt i.e. potassium or sodium metabisulphite. Being highly soluble, it ensures better mixing and is an effective preservative. It prevents darkening of pared fruits and vegetables due to enzymatic action. It can't be used in products stored in tin cans because it causes pin holes in metals and forms ugly incrustation in the form of tin sulphide. It is used at 0.6g/kg of the finished product.

(vi) **Sorbic acid:** It is an organic acid having antimicrobial properties. Its level of use in jams, fruit syrups and pastes is 0.025, 0.02 and 0.10-0.20%, respectively. Sodium and potassium salts of sorbic acid are used as fungistatic agents for foods specially on the surface and in the wrapping materials.

(vii) **Radiation:** Ionizing radiations (Alpha, beta particles and gamma rays) are used in preservation of selected food products. Their safety for human consumption has to be made fool-proof. However, the economics and other aspects of its application have to be worked out to make it more popular.

(viii) **Antibiotics:** An antibiotic is a chemical substance produced by microorganisms which have the capacity of inhibiting growth or destroying other kinds of microorganisms. Subtelin (antibiotic obtained from *Bacillus subtilis*) is used to facilitate preservation of asparagus, corn and peas (canned products) at 10 to 20 ppm levels. Nisin (antibiotic produced by *Streptococcus lactis*) is widely used in the food industry in canned food. It is more commonly used in canning of mushrooms, tomatoes and milk products (acid foods). Nisin suppresses the growth of spoilage organisms mainly the gas producing, spore forming bacteria and toxin producing *Clostridium botulinum*.

Practical Hints on Food Storage

Dry grains and products Dry products should have optimum moisture of 10% in tropical climate for safe storage. Cereals are dried completely, packed in air tight bins, gunny bags, earthenware pots etc. and stored in a cool and dry place. Polished-rice has better keeping quality than hand-pounded rice. Whole wheat flour, maida keep well for 1-2 months. For preventing infestation of semolina, it can be roasted lightly and stored in air-tight containers.

Chapatis will stay fresh if kept in an air-tight container after cooling to room temperature. Application of butter oil on the chapati will help to retain the freshness for longer period.

Bread and other baked products must be allowed to cool completely before storing. For maintaining freshness, wrap them in a cellophane cover and keep them in the refrigerator.

Milk: Fresh milk must be boiled, cooled and stored in a refrigerator in a covered container. Milk exposed to sunlight loses riboflavin and ascorbic acid and flavour of the milk deteriorates in a short time.

Meat, chicken & fish: All these are wrapped loosely in wax paper or cellophane and frozen. Freezing is one of the best methods of preserving fresh flavour, colour, texture and eating quality. They may be thawed in the refrigerator before cooking. Never refreeze the thawed meat as it spoils its texture.

Eggs: For the best quality, eggs should be kept in the refrigerator. They should be placed so that the broad ends of the eggs are up, thus preventing movement of the Yolk.

Fruits: Fruits continue to respire after harvesting, i.e., they take O_2 and give off CO_2. Cold temperature reduces the fruit metabolism and ripening processes. All fruits should be washed before being placed in the refrigerator. Citrus fruits can be kept fresh longer by keeping them in polythene covers. Ripened bananas are not stored at low temperature because of a colour change in the skin.

Vegetables: These can preserved for longer periods with freshness by keeping them in a refrigerator after wrapped in a polythene cover. Green leafy vegetables are washed and drained thoroughly; then they are packed in polythene cover and stored in refrigerator. Roots and tubers including carrot, beetroot, potatoes and mature onions can be stored in a cool, dark and dry place where there is circulation of air.

Storage of Manufactured Feed

Keep the manufactured diet under cool and dry conditions: The enemies of dry food are oxygen, light, heat, and moisture. Thus, keeping the diet in opaque, airtight containers and under cool and dry conditions is essential to long-term storage.

Prevent potential contamination from biological sources and chemical contaminants: Measures should be taken to prevent potential contamination by bird, rodent, or insect infestations. Diets should be stored away from any drugs, pesticides, or other potential contaminants.

Avoid post-processing contamination: Most instances of microbial contamination are the result of recontamination after processing. As dry food exits the extruder, it has reached temperatures sufficient to destroy pathogenic organism. However, since it may be in contact with non-sterile equipment or materials prior to packaging, it may not remain microorganism-free even in an unopened bag. Most of the animals normally tolerate small doses of even pathogenic microorganisms. However in feeding 'specific pathogen-free' animals extra care is needed to avoid potential exposure.

Appropriate storage of feed: A small degree of contamination may present a potential problem only if the conditions provide for microbial growth (e.g. moisture, heat). This emphasizes the need for appropriate storage of food, as well as proper handling of food and sanitation of utensils and facilities.

Sterilization of diets for specific pathogen-free and especially germ-free animals: Dry diets can be autoclaved or exposed to irradiation to achieve sterility, but only after additional consideration has been given in formulating diets to potential nutrient losses due to the sterilization procedures. Nutrients that are generally synthesized by gut flora in the normal animal (e.g. biotin, vitamin K) are typically added to most commercial petfoods. Extra care must be given to the adequate provision of these substances in diets intended for germ-free colonies.

Due diligence should be exercised to ensure that sterilized foods are not exposed to potential contaminants till they are consumed.

Canned food is sterile and hermetically sealed and so they retain the wholesomeness and nutritive values. Extreme temperature conditions (especially freezing), rough handling or any other action that might dent or rupture the cans should be avoided. Once canned food has been opened, the risk of contamination with potentially pathogenic organisms greatly increases.

17

Metabolic Problems in Wild Animals - Wildlife Diseases

Metabolic Disorders

The diseases associated with imbalance in 'input' of dietary nutrients and 'output' from animal products (like foetus production, milk, etc.) is clubbed under metabolic disorders. These problems are less recorded than that actually occurs in wild animals. The nutritional status of wild animals determines their well-being, their maximal production and infant survivability and resistance to environmental changes, infectious and parasitic diseases.

Metabolic processes are greatly strained during winter in both the sexes and starvation is not uncommon in deers particularly in small individuals on over-browsed range. On the contrary, feed intake increases in spring season as the feed supply remains no longer deficient and the body weight increases.

Impact of Carbohydrates on Health Status of Wild Mammals

Ketosis or acetonemia in wild ruminants

This is common in wild ruminants (giraffe, deer, antelope, wild goat, wild sheep and wild bovid). Carbohydrates are the main energy sources of herbivore and omnivore wild mammals. The energy required is more in young growing mammals and the mammals in the advanced stage of pregnancy. Herbivorous ruminants are dependent on only coarse roughage such as dry grass hay and straw, which are very poor sources to supply all the energy needs.

234

The dietary carbohydrates are fermented in the rumen to short chain fatty acids (acetate in majority amount, propionate in moderate amount and butyrate in lesser amount). Hence, the glucose needs are largely met by gluconeogenesis and it is to be understood that propionate and amino acids are the major precursors for gluconeogenesis. But due to carbohydrate, mainly starch insufficiency, oxaloacetate is not available for the entry of acetyl Co A into TCA cycle. Hence, animals develop ketosis due to negative energy balance and animals come to use fat depot for energy sources.

Ketosis may also result in those wild mammals (mainly ruminants) which are on starvation for several days (aetiology may be due to unavailability of feed or atonicity of rumen or recurrent ruminal impaction or other ruminal atony associated with some primary illness). Ketosis in wild ruminants is characterized by (a) ketonemia (b) ketonurea (c) ketolactea (d) hypoglycemia (e) poor liver glycogen content. The syndrome is based on gradual but moderate decrease in appetite over 2-4 days with a rapid decrease in body weight and a characteristic odour of ketone bodies (sweet to vinegar smell).

Pregnancy Toxaemia in Sheep and Goats

Hypoglycemic syndrome is also common in wild sheep and goats. This is also known as pregnancy toxaemia, a form of ketosis. It has been observed that these wild sheep and goats have been fed poor quality roughages and grasses. Twinning in sheep and goats increases the rate of occurrence of pregnancy toxaemia. Ketosis can be diagnosed on the basis of clinical signs, ketone bodies presence in urine or in milk or by reduced blood pH.

Treatment includes to increase blood glucose level giving glucose intravenously or ringer's lactate intravenously, oral feeding of glycerol or propylene glycol, oral feeding of sodium propionate, hormonal therapy - betamethasone, triaminolone, prednisolone and anabolic steroids (dinapol and trienbolone).

Neonatal Hypoglycemia in Wild Animals

This occurs mainly due to insufficient intake of colostrum or milk from mother due to multiple reasons and this causes metabolic derangements. Hypoglycemia occurs in the affected wild animal species. The symptoms include pale skin, weakness, recumbency, hypothermia, incoordination with terminal convulsions. Monitoring the infant for proper feeding (ensure for proper energy intake) and monitoring of the mother on proper nursing may help for the prevention of this problem in case of wild animals.

Parturient Paresis (milk fever) in Wild Ruminants

This condition can be anticipated in wild cervids in the newly fawned deer or antelopes that have given birth. This can be anticipated especially when there are twin births. Milk fever may affect surely the gaur, mithun, etc. ruminants. This condition commonly occurs within two days of parturition and this may also occur few weeks before or after the parturition. Hypocalcemia coupled with hypomagnesemia may be the cause.

Lactation Tetany in Wild Equids

This can be anticipated in case of wild equids reared under captive conditions. Zebras, wild asses and wild horses may get affected by this condition and often, it occurs in the lactating equids, either at about 10th day, after giving birth. Even after the prolonged transport or after the severe exertion, this condition may occur.

Colic

Colic is more commonly encountered in case of elephants in severe metabolic derangements like acidosis. Several factors may precipitate the colic condition in general. These include feeding of unaccustomed food material, excess feeding of the routine food materials, obstruction anywhere in the gastrointestinal tract, lesser exercise, non-provision of adequate amounts of water for the drinking purposes.

Hypothyroidism in Captive Wild Mammals

Deficiency of iodine may occur in any species of wild mammals. Obesity, alopecia, dullness with lethargic movements and lowered serum cholesterol are the major features in this hypothyroidism.

Metabolic bone Diseases

Bone diseases associated with metabolic disorders are comparatively more common in wild animals.

Rickets

Failure of mineralization of bone matrix in young, growing animals results in rickets.

Osteoporsis

It is a state of bone in which resorption of osteoid overbalances the deposition of new tissue. The net result is the decrease in the organic matrix of the bone and thus, density of the bone. Protein deficiency also may have some influencing effect on the occurrence of osteoporosis. Osteoporosis occurs in both the adults and juveniles, where the already hardened bones become weakened by the withdrawal of calcium for metabolic purposes. Senile osteoporosis is also recorded in old wild mammals.

Osteomalacia

Insufficient mineralization of osteoids leads to softening of bones and decreased bone density. The condition is seen in adult bones in which mineralization fail to keep pace with mineral resorption. Bone eaters like hyaena if deprived of bones in their diet may end up in this bone disorder.

Fibrous Osteodystrophy

Mineral imbalances or osteoporosis causes osteoclastic resorption of osteoids and it is being replaced by highly cellular connective tissue. Bones of face and mandible is frequently affected although conditions may involve other bones. Deposition of connective tissue is a compensatory mechanism for structural weakness resulting from softening of the bones. Clinical signs include enlargement of facial and mandibular bones. Dysponea results due to occlusion of nasal passage. Prehension and mastication becomes difficult.

Osteomalacia and osteodystrophy are caused by feeding diet with less calcium (provision of minced meat, liver and heart without bone or with less bone), failure in proper absorption of calcium (due to diseases of gastrointestinal tract / excessive phosphorus in diet), insufficient calcium supplement and hormonal imbalances, lack of vitamin D especially in indoor-kept wild animals and prolonged storage of the ration (since it may lead to less vitamin D_3).

Metabolic bone disease in bears: This disease has been observed in bears fed meat-diet. If ground muscle meat is fed to captive bears, calcium carbonate should be supplemented @ 400 mg/100g of meat, in addition to multivitamin-trace mineral supplement. Hypothyroidism has been reported in a grizzly bear that was thought to be on a diet low in iodine which contained goitrogenic substances in the form of nitrates.

Problems Anticipated due to Abrupt Change of Diet in Wild Animals

Abrupt change of diet in amounts and ratio of concentrate and roughage or ingredients of diets is a recurring cause of health problems in animals. Small ruminants have relatively fast metabolism compared to larger ruminant livestock and tend to eat more frequently. Therefore, a large meal once or twice daily consisting of a large concentration of grain is somewhat unnatural and makes small ruminants susceptible to metabolic diseases. Digestive systems of small ruminants are sensitive and require time to adapt to changes in rations. When dietary changes are made over a time, it allows the microbial populations in the rumen to shift and adapt to the type of feedstuff being offered.

A rapid shift to a high grain ration may cause enterotoxaemia, cause animals to refuse feed, or induce diarrhoea or other digestive upset. Similarly, when a small ruminant that is accustomed to consuming a high grain ration is suddenly introduced to forage only diet, the rumen microbes are unable to digest the fibrous portions of the diet effectively. Changing rations gradually and allowing time for adaptation is important for good health of the animal and assures continued productivity. This practice applies to all animals including birds.

Wildlife Diseases

Wildlife Diseases Pose a Risk to Small Ruminants and Their Farmers

Infectious pathogens from wild animals have become increasingly important in recent years, as they have had a substantial impact in livestock and human health. A large number of pathogens are zoonotic and can infect multiple animal species. Multi-host pathogens are predominant among animal and human emerging diseases. Of 800 zoonotic diseases currently identified, 77% are caused by pathogens that affect wildlife; of 125 emerging zoonotic diseases, 90% affect wildlife. Of the diseases that have emerged in the last few decades around 75% are of wildlife origin (Billinis, 2013). Many factors influence changes in diseases incidence. Close interaction of humans and livestock with wild animals has led to increased frequency of zoonotic infections. It is reported that wildlife may be carriers of several pathogens, which can be transmitted to domestic small ruminants and their farmers.

Mycobacterium bovis is both the causative agent of bovine tuberculosis (TB) and a zoonotic pathogen. In humans, considerably fewer cases of TB are caused by *M.bovis* than *M. tuberculosis*. The routes of transmission from animals to humans are well known and include direct exposure to infected animals or consumption of contaminated animal products.

Bovine Tuberculosis

Transmission of bovine tuberculosis (*Mycobacterium bovis*) among wildlife (elk and white tailed deer) and livestock has created important risks for conservation and agriculture. Chronic wasting disease (CWD) is prevalent in wild white-tailed deer population. Deer population control has been suggested to reduce the prevalence of CWD.

M. bovis is the cause of tuberculosis in a wide array of domesticated and wild animals, and it remains a major veterinary health problem worldwide, causing severe economic losses from livestock disease, death and export restrictions. Humans become infected by ingesting raw milk or undercooked meat, or by the aerosol route from infected animals (animal-to-human) or humans (human-to-human). In developed countries, pasteurization and test-and-slaughter methods have controlled the disease, and zoonotic infections are relatively rare, accounting for only 0.3-7.2% of tuberculosis cases. In developing countries (which do not practice control measures) the disease is more common, although few data on prevalence exist (as cited by Monath, 2013).

Wild animals are a major source of infection of *M. bovis* among domestic livestock (Humblet et al., 2009). Measures aimed at control of *M. bovis* by culling wildlife reservoirs are problematic, with inconsistent results and ethical concerns. Vaccination of wildlife is an attractive alternative control measure, especially since the traditional tuberculosis vaccine (Bacille Calmette-Guerin, BCG) derived from *M. bovis* is effective when orally administered. Examples of wildlife that serve as maintenance hosts of *M. bovis* and sources of infection in livestock, include white-tail deer, wild boar, red and fallow deer, badgers, African buffalo (*Syncerus caffer*) and brushtail possums (*Trichosurus vulpecula*). Brushtail possums in New Zealand have been experimentally vaccinated using oral BCG and shown to be resistant to challenge with *M. bovis*. Vaccine efficacy against naturally acquired tuberculosis was 95-96%. Collins, D.M. et al. (2007; Vaccine 25:4659) concluded that oral vaccination of possums could be a practical strategy contributing to elimination of M. bovis in livestock.

Wildlife and Paratuberculosis

Paratuberculosis (Johne's disease) is infectious granulomatous enteritis caused by *Mycobacterium avium paratuberculosis* (MAP). Currently there are still no ideal, cost-effective methods for the control of paratuberculosis in domestic ruminants. The existence of wildlife reservoirs of MAP might also comes in way of the eradication of disease. The intensification of deer farming in Europe and worldwide has increased the prevalence of paratuberculosis in these ruminants. The high MAP prevalence in farmed deer could potentially contaminate wildlife populations, if infected are released, since MAP has demonstrated its ability to infect a wide range of wild ruminant species, including wild cervids, wild bovids, non-ruminant wild species and carnivores. Carta et al. (2013) showed evidence that MAP circulates almost worldwide among a diversity of wild vertebrates including ruminant and non-ruminant species. The likelihood of MAP (in wildlife) interference with TB diagnosis must be considered in attempts to monitor TB in wildlife.

Wildlife - Livestock Interface

Foot and Mouth disease (FMD): FMD affects cloven-hoofed animals, including domestic and wild bovines. When the FMD affected ruminants or pigs entered a reserve forest, chances of the disease spreading among wildlife such as Indian bison, elephants, spotted deer and sambar are very high.

The genus Salmonella is found throughout the world and is a potential pathogen for most vertebrates. It is also the most common cause of food-borne illness in humans, and wildlife is an emerging source of food-borne disease in humans due to the consumption of game meat. Wild boar is one of the most abundant European game species and these wild swine are known to be carriers of zoonotic and food-borne pathogens such as Salmonella.

Impact of Baiting and Supplemental Feeding of Wildlife on the Risk of Transmission of Infectious Diseases

Baiting and supplemental feeding of Wildlife result in large congregations of individuals and species in a small area. The risk of intra-species and inter-species disease transmission likely increases in such situations. Baiting and supplemental feeding of wildlife are widespread, yet highly controversial management practices, with important implications for ecosystems, livestock production, and potentially human health (Sorensen et al., 2013)

Supplemental feed is provided to wildlife to address various ecological and socio-economic purposes such as alleviating mortality in winter season, increasing reproductive success, controlling wildlife damage to crops and the environment, reducing wildlife-vehicle collisions, controlling animal migration routes, and optimizing tourism opportunities.

Baiting: Baiting involves the purposeful placement of natural or artificial food resources in order to attract and /or retain wildlife in an area to capture them for research purpose, to capture, vaccinate, and / or treatment of animals for control of infectious diseases and vectors.

Supplemental feeding: Supplemental feeding is the provision of food by humans with the intention to enhance some specific physical characteristics of individuals or to benefit population dynamics, e.g., increased antler growth, fecundity and survival. Winter feeding is as specific type of supplemental feeding to compensate for lower natural food availability for wildlife and higher energetic demands during winter conditions, primarily to prevent starvation mortalities and maintain body condition. Intercept or diversionary feeding is the provision of food at strategic places to modify animal distribution and movements so as to reduce environmental damage, to divert wildlife away from major vehicle traffic corridors to reduce animal-vehicle collisions, or prevent disease transmission among wildlife and livestock.

Sorensen et al. (2013) provided a comprehensive review of the scientific evidence of baiting and supplemental feeding on disease transmission risk in wildlife, with an emphasis on large herbivores in North America. In North America specifically, concerns have been raised regarding the ecological and economic impacts of such feeding practices following the emergence of chronic wasting disease (CWD) in free-ranging and domestic elk (*Cervus canadensis*), mule deer (*Odocoileus hemionus hemionus*), black-tailed deer (*Odocoileus hemionus columbianus*), white-tailed deer (*Odocoileus virginianus*), and moose (*Alces alces*), and outbreaks of bovine tuberculosis and brucellosis in elk and white-tailed deer.

Transmission of infectious diseases: Large congregations of wildlife around feeding or baiting sites have been widely implicated as a major mechanism increasing the risk of both direct and indirect transmission of infectious diseases and spread. Infectious diseases include bovine tuberculosis (a bacterial disease that occurs in wildlife and livestock throughout the world), bovine brucellosis (a chronic bacterial disease caused by *Brucella abortus*, and is found in livestock and wildlife populations around the world), chronic wasting disease, psoroptic mange or scabies in elk, skin papillomas and fibromas (skin tumours) in ungulates (deer, moose, caribou and pronghorn).

Chronic wasting disease (CWD) is a neurological disease belonging to the group of transmissible spongiform encephalopathies (TSEs). In contrast with other TSEs, such as bovine spongiform encephalopathy in cattle or scrapie in sheep, CWD is currently known to only infect free-ranging and domestic elk, mule deer, black-tailed deer, white-tailed deer, and moose (Edmunds, 2008). CWD is both infectious and contagious (Williams et al., 2002) but specific details on the pathways of transmission remain poorly understood (Miller et al., 2006).

Direct transmission: If one or more individuals are carrying an infectious organism or prion, its transmission to uninfected individuals may be facilitated by higher rates of contact between animals gathered at a single site (Miller et al., 1998). Direct transmission is especially problematic in social species, such as elk and deer, as contact occurs frequently and regularly within familial social groups. In addition, crowding of wildlife in confined spaces has also been shown to induce stress responses, which can reduce immune function and increase disease susceptibility (Forristal et al., 2012).

Indirect transmission: Disease transmission can also occur when animals consume feed, water, and associated soil contaminated by the urine, blood, nasal secretions, saliva, or faeces from infectious individuals. Risks of infection increase when multiple individuals and species congregate in a confined area, such as bait sites or feeding stations. The specific route and risk of disease transmission is, in part, dependent on the biology of the specific pathogen.

Implications for human and livestock health: Diseases in wildlife pose serious risk to human and livestock health. Baiting and feeding may play an important role in facilitating the maintenance and spread of disease. Evidence for this is found for bovine TB in white-tailed deer and for brucellosis in elk. Nevertheless, most scientific studies on the role of baiting and feeding on disease occurrence and transmission do not compare prevalence between fed and unfed individuals or populations, which then become mere observations of disease prevalence at feeding grounds (Sorensen et al., 2013). It is also reported that majority of emerging infectious diseases found in humans come from wildlife.

The decision to implement feeding or baiting as a wildlife management tool should at least consider the strong potential for disease transmission and spread. If feeding or baiting is indeed to be followed, Sorensen et al. (2013) recommended a pro-active approach to limit disease transmission through a combination of preventive actions such as low density feeding, vaccination if possible, and continuous monitoring of disease prevalence.

Licensing from Municipality

Municipality has to issue license to dogs, elephants etc (within its jurisdiction) to ensure veterinary public health and to see that hygiene is maintained. The criteria include (for elephants) deworming at every six months, a TB test once in two years, changing the sand in the enclosure and whitewashing the entire enclosure once in six months.

One Health Initiative

One Health Initiative seeks to establish "collaborative efforts of multiple disciplines working locally, nationally and globally to attain optimal health for people, animals and our environment (AVMA, 2008).

Zoonotic diseases refer to those diseases transmissible from animals to humans. Certain zoonotic diseases have the potential for pandemic spread by human contagion, such as avian influenza, SARS and the Middle East Respiratory Syndrome coronavirus. It is estimated that 56 different zoonotic diseases are responsible annually for 2.5 billion cases of human disease with 2.7 million deaths and substantial reductions in livestock production (Grace et al., 2012). Animals, including livestock and companion animals, also suffer illness and death following infection with many zoonotic infections, and livestock and poultry are subject to large-scale intentional destruction as a means of preventing human infections, resulting in huge economic losses. Wild animals, including endangered species, may also be mortally affected.

Causative agents of zoonotic diseases: Causative agents of zoonotic diseases, including viruses, parasites, bacteria, fungi, and prions, have extraordinarily varied lifecycles and modes of transmission. Some may persist between periods of active transmission in soil or invertebrate species. Many have silent transmission cycles involving wild animals that have co-evolved with the infectious agent and exhibit no signs of disease. Some zoonotic diseases occur when a causative agent harbored by a wild animal reservoir jumps species to domesticated animals and thence to humans. Others are primarily diseases of domesticated animal species.

Humans may be infected by direct contact with wild or domesticated animals, or indirectly by ingestion of contaminated milk or meat, inhalation of aerosolized secretions or excreta, fomites, or hematophagous insect or tick vectors. Despite this complexity of epidemiological patterns, the opportunities for intervention often boil down to a few simple bottlenecks in the transmission process. For example, milk-borne diseases can be prevented by pasteurization, certain meat-borne diseases by inspection and animal husbandry improvements (e.g., trichinella, bovine tuberculosis), and other diseases avoided by limiting contact with known high risk species (e.g., tularemia, turtle-borne salmonellosis, exposure to bats carrying henipaviruses).

Frameworks for vaccine-based interventions: Vaccines are an important means of prevention and control of zoonotic infectious diseases in humans and domesticated animals. Three major epidemiological frameworks are identified for the control of zoonotic disease by means of vaccination of animals (Monath, T.P., 2013).

Framework I vaccines are used for protection of humans and economically valuable animals, where neither plays a role in the transmission cycle; one example (West Nile vaccine) of a single product developed for use in animals and humans.

Framework II vaccines are indicated for domesticated animals as a means of preventing disease in both animals and humans. The agents of concern are transmitted directly or indirectly (e.g. via arthropod vectors) from animals to humans. A number of examples of the use of Framework II vaccines are provided, e.g. against anthrax, brucellosis, *Escherischia coli* O157, rabies, Rift Valley fever, Venezuelan equine encephalitis, and Hendra virus disease. Vaccination of domesticated animals has the potential to protect humans against these zoonoses.

Framework III vaccines are used to immunize wild animals as a means of preventing transmission of disease agents to humans and domesticated animals. Wild animals play a major role in transmission of the disease to humans and domestic animals. Most zoonotic diseases are maintained in transmission cycles involving wild mammals or birds. However, because of the difficulties in vaccinating specific host species, wildlife immunization as a means of preventing spread to domestic animals and humans has been applied in only a few diseases. Examples are reservoir-targeted, oral bait rabies, Mycobacterium bovis and Lyme disease (most common vector-borne disease in USA) vaccines. Some interventions based on the immunization of animals could lead to rapid and relatively inexpensive advances in public health.

See also Appendix for information on Rabies.

18

Feeding of Common Birds and Pet Birds

Pet Animal or Pet Bird

A pet is an animal kept for companionship and enjoyment. Pet animal is a household animal, as opposed to livestock, laboratory animals, working animals or sport animals, which are kept for economic reasons.

The most popular pets are noted for their loyalty, for their attractive appearance, or for their song. Pets also generally seem to provide their owners some health benefits. Keeping pets has been shown to help relieve stress. Walking a dog can provide both the owner and the dog with exercise, fresh air, and social interaction. Pet animals vary from dog, cat, horse, lovebirds, pigeons, fishes, amphibians, rodents etc.

Common Pet Birds

Various species of birds are maintained by pet bird lovers. The hobby of bird keeping offers considerable potential, ranging from enjoying budgerigar to keeping tame duck on a garden pond. Common pet birds are Bengalese finches, parrots, lovebirds, pigeons and doves, bantams and other fowls and pheasants and quail.

Growth of vegetation of all types offering a green canopy and fruit bearing trees and grain crops cultivated in the area has increased the insect population. These features generally attract the bird population. Some common birds sighted in the veterinary college, Puducherry premises (Sreekumar et al., 2011) are mentioned in the Table 1. Most of the birds belong to order Passerformes and the families include corvidae, pittidae, dicrurudae, sturnidae, estreldidae, passeridae, camphiphagiidae and monarchidae.

244

Table 1: Common birds sighted in Veterinary College premises*

Common name	Scientific name	Order	Family
House crow	*Corvus splendens*	Passeriformes	Corvidae
Jungle crow	*Corvus macrorhynchos*	Passeriformes	Corvidae
Indian treepie	*Dendrocitta vagabunda*	Passeriformes	Corvidae
Indian pitta	*Pitta brachyura*	Passeriformes	Pittidae
Black drongo	*Dicrurus macrocercus*	Passeriformes	Dicrurudae
Common myna	*Acridotheres tristis*	Passeriformes	Sturnidae
Spotted munia	*Lonchra punctulata*	Passeriformes	Estreldidae
Black-headed munia	*L.malacca*	Passeriformes	Estreldidae
House sparrow	*Passer domesticus*	Passeriformes	Passeridae
Small minivet	*Pericrocotus cinnamomeus*	Passeriformes	Camphiphagiidae
Asian paradise-flycatcher	*Terpsiphone paradise*	Passeriformes	Monarchidae
Grey francolin	*Francolinus pondicerianus*	Galliformes	Phasianidae
Indian peafowl	*Pavo cristatus*	Galliformes	Phasianidae
Common hoopoe	*Upupa epops*	Upupiformes	Upupidae
Small blue kingfisher	*Alcedo atthis*	Coraciiformes	Alcedinidae
Pied crested cuckoo	*Clamater jacobinus*	Cuculiformes	Cuculidae
Drongo cuckoo	*Surniculus lugubris*	Cuculiformes	Centropodidae
Rose-ringed parakeet	*Psittacula krameri*	Psittaciformes	Psittacidae
Asian palm swift	*Cypsiurus balasiensis*	Apodiformes	Apodidae
Eastern grass owl	*Tyto longimembris*	Strigiformes	Tytonidae
Blue rock pigeon	*Columbia livia*	Columbiformes	Columbidae
Spotted dove	*Streptopelia chinensis*	Columbiformes	Columbidae
Shikra	*Accipiter badius*	Falconiformes	Accipitridae

*Sreekumar et al. (2011)

Order Passeriformes and Family Estreldidae

Munias

Lonchura is a genus of the Estreldidae finch family, and includes munias (or minias), mannikins, and silverbills. They are resident breeding birds in Africa and in South Asia from India and Sri Lanka east to Indonesia and the Philippine. The species in this genus are similar in size and structure, with stubby bills, stocky bodies and long tails. Most are 10-12 cm in length.

Plumage is usually a combination of browns, black and white, with the sexes similar, but duller and less contrasted for immature birds.

There are different species like black headed munia (*Lonchura Malacca*), white backed munia, spotted munia (*Lonchura punctulata*). Munias are very popular as cage birds. During the breeding season the cock sings weakly for his mate. Munias are very sociable birds. The nest is a large domed grass structure into which 4-10 white eggs are laid. Some species also build communal roosting nests for overnight rest. They are small gregarious birds which feed mainly on seeds, usually in relatively open habitats, preferring to feed on the ground or on reeds and grasses. Several species have been noted to feed on algae such as Spirogyra.

Munia, a small colourful melodious finch, nests in bushes and shrub, is losing its habitat all over the country much like the house sparrow.

Bengalese Finches

The Bengalese (or society) finches are probably derived from the white-backed munia (*Lonchura striata*). These small birds are about 4 inches long. The white-backed munia is found in India and Sri Lanka. It is primarily brown with very dark, almost black, head and breast; the rump and underside are white.

The birds of this particular group are categorized by their dependence on seed as a major item in their diet. Thus they are described as 'hardbills' possessing beaks able to crack seeds and dehusking them before swallowing the inner kernel. These birds do not become tame or learn to talk like parrots and certain softbills. Many species will nest, however, either indoors or in garden aviaries and can be accommodated together successfully in mixed groups. Finches ranks among the least expensive and most freely available birds.

Parrots and Parakeets

The order Psittaciformes (family Psittacidae) consists of approximately three hundred and thirty species, which are mainly confined to tropical regions. The term parakeets generally applies to long tailed slender bird belonging to the family Psittacidae. The genus *Psittacula* is made up of the larger parakeets and the males have red beaks. The genus *Psittacula* is made up of the larger parakeets and the males have red beaks. In India there is no parrot but only parakeets (parrot like birds). The common parakeets are budgerigars, rose-ringed parakeet (*Psitacula krameri*), blossom headed parakeet or plum head parakeet and blue winged parakeet or bamboo parakeet or malabar parakeet. Parakeets, if acquired young can learn to talk quite well and they will develop elaborate vocabulary.

They have sharply curved upper beak that fits over their lower bill. The degree of curvature depends on the species concerned, and this in turn reflects its function. Long billed Corella uses its upper mandible to dig for roots.

Another well-known characteristic of parrots is their potentially long lifespan. The parrots have the ability to mimic the sounds, including that of human voice. Parrots obtained in young can be easily tamed and devoted to their owners.

Lovebirds

Lovebirds are a group of small short tailed parrots occurring in Africa and on certain offshore islands. Lovebirds are very hardy and long-lived. They make excellent pets and tame readily if obtained at a young age; older birds may become aggressive. Determining the sex of lovebirds is difficult.

All love birds are characterized by their unusual breeding behaviour. Love birds collect nesting materials, with which they line the nest site, carrying it either in their beak or tucked in among the feather of the rump, depending upon the species concerned. They are highly attractive and rewarding bird to keep.

Budgerigar

The budgerigar or common pet parakeet (*Melopsittacus undulatus*), often called a budgie or parakeet, is a small parrot and the only species in the Australian genus Melopsittacus.

Cockatiel

Cockatiel is another member of the parrot family from the arid interior Australia. The distinctive crest of the cockatiel can be held erect or lowered, which is a feature otherwise peculiar to the cockatoos. Nevertheless, unlike cockatoos, cockatiel has evolved a long tail and is of slimmer proportion overall. They also have very different call notes, cockatiels possess an inoffensive voice, compared with the harsh screeches of the cockatoos.

Cockatoos

All cockatoos can be instantly recognized by their crests, which are raised when the birds are excited or alarmed. Most cockatoos are white but some are pink or black. They have extremely strong, heavy bills. The largest is the Black Palm cockatoo of 28 inches. The Sulphur-crested Cockatoo (Cacatua galerita) is a relatively large white cockatoo found in wooded habitats in Australia and New Guinea. They are well known in aviculture, although they can be demanding pets.

Macaw

Macaw is characterized by large area of essentially bare facial skin on either side of the head. Though they posses fearsome beaks, macaws can prove very gentle. But never take any chance with an unknown bird. They are not usually mimics, but are certainly intelligent birds. Macaws show a strong tendency to become one-person pets, and this can present a great problem when purchasing a tame adult bird that is used to its surrounding. They have long potential lifespan and mature slowly.

Pigeons and Doves (order Columbiformes and family Columbidae)

The pigeons and doves have fairly uniform appearance. The term 'dove' tends to be reserved for smaller birds, but this does not apply in every instance. Most species eat seed, but a few genera subsist largely on fruit. Examples: Blue rock pigeon (*Columba livea*), spotted Dove (*Streptopelia chinensis*) and fancy pigeons; Emerald dove or Bronze-winged dove is a strict forest dweller and is part of all the wooded areas of the Nilgiris and feed on fallen seeds and berries.

Koels (order Cuculiformes and family Cuculidae)

The true koels (Eudynamys) are a genus of Cuckoos from Asia, Australia and the Pacific. They are large sexually dimorphic cuckoos which eat fruits and insects and have loud distinctive calls. They are brood parasites, laying their eggs in the nests of other species. Cuckoos have the habit of laying eggs in crow's nest and the bird catchers mistake the cuckoo for a crow chick (Cuckoo are covered under Schedule 4 of the Wildlife Protection Act, 1972). In New Zealand the Long-tailed koel is known as the Long-tailed cuckoo. Drongo cuckoo (*Surniculus lugubris*) belongs to Centropodidae family.

Two other species, the White-crowned koel and the Dwarf koel, are also known as koels but are in their own monotypic genera. The male is all black, about the same size but slimmer than the crow. The female is brown, profusely spotted and barred with white. Male's loud sound is monotonus calls kuo kuo kuo and the female has metallic clicking call which carries a long way.

Bantams

Bantams are small fowls, which are in some instance, have larger counterparts, such as the Rhode Island Red. They are valued as foster parents, being capable of hatching the eggs for waterfowls, pheasants and similar birds. Bantams clutch a variety of eggs from quail up to two goose eggs, and are known as fearsome mothers, with a high success rate in rearing any egg hatched.

The light breeds of bantam are generally active and lively. Heavy breeds of bantam tend to prove the best broodiness. These include the Australorps, which are black in colour and Marans which lay brown eggs. Fancy breed is the third category that is primarily kept for their decorative appearance. These include the Polish, Silkie, Frizzle etc.

Bantams have become increasingly popular as pets as well as for show purposes because they are smaller and have more varied and exotic colours and feather patterns than other chickens. They are suitable for smaller backyards as they do not need as much space as other breeds.

Bantam hens are also used as laying hens, although bantam eggs are only about one-half to one-third the size of a regular hen egg. The bantam chicken eats the same foods as a normal chicken.

Pheasants and Quail

These birds spent much of their time on the ground and although some can be kept satisfactorily at liberty, the majority is housed in aviary surrounding. Grass provides a natural base for an aviary, and will be eaten by most birds in this group. They will often spend considerable period of time walking close to the perimeter of the aviary, it is often recommended to construct paths of sand around the end and plant up the central area. Examples for quails are bobwhite quail, Gambel's quail, Japanese quail.

Pheasants are maintained as aviary birds in their own right. They are not suitable for being kept indoor, unless their enclosure is usually spacious. Pheasants are characterized by strong sexual dimorphism, males being highly ornate with bright colours and adornments such as wattles and long tails. Males are usually larger than females and have longer tails. Males play no part in rearing the young. Pheasants typically eat seeds and some insects.

Feeding of Birds

Omnivores and Oligivores

The term omnivore (polyvore) is most appropriate for species that consume both animal and plant foods. Oligivore refers to specialist feeder. In the wild, the exact choice is determined by a combination of factors, including: seasonal availability of food, foraging efficiency, changing nutrient requirements, palatability and predator patterns. Many omnivorous species fit into one of the oligivore categories seasonally or during some phase of their life history.

Classifications of birds based on their primary feed (Table 2; trophic-level classification) are herbivore, insectivore, frugivore, nectarivore, piscivore, folivore, granivore, fungivore, etc. Faunivores are birds that consume foods almost exclusively of animal origin while florivores consume plant matter. Birds (geese and swan) that consume primarily grasses are graminivores. Many birds select the components of the plant that have the highest concentration of digestible nutrients, such as that found in grain, fruit, or nectar, and are granivores, frugivores, and nectarivores, respectively. Birds that probe or drill for the saps, gums, or resins in plants are known as exudativores. Birds (flamingos) that filter or select zooplankton from the water are known as planktonivores. The sharp-beaked Ground Finch found on one of the islands of the Galapagos is described as a sanguinivore because it consumes blood from other birds as a primary food item.

However, these terms that describe the consumption categories are not acceptable to botanists and ecologists. For example, to a botanist frugivores should include all birds that eat the fertile ovaries of plants and their associated structures. Many ecologists consider this term too vague and consider those birds that disperse seeds, and thereby aid in plant reproduction, as 'true frugivores' while those birds that destroy seeds by digesting them are considered as granivores. Nutritionally, frugivores eat soft, moist fruits, which are relatively nutrient-dilute, whereas granivores eat hard, dry, nutrient-dense fruits (e.g., beans, nuts), regardless of the plant family of origin.

Common Dietary Ingredients

Most bird diets consist of seeds (seed-eaters; granivores), except for the fruit and nectar-consuming birds. Some birds consume seeds and dry nuts (seed and nut-eaters). Seeds consumed by the birds are of two types: cereal grains and legume and oil seeds. Cereal grains contain a higher proportion of carbohydrates. Examples of cereal grains (and millets) are paddy/rice, wheat, maize, dehusked oat kernels, sorghum, bajra and small millets. Legume seeds are cowpea, pea, bengal gram or chick pea, etc. Oil seeds are high in fat and low in carbohydrates. Examples of oil seeds are sunflower seeds, peanuts, safflower, rape, niger and linseed.

Both cereal grains and oil seeds are purchased, cleaned from the dust and dirt and mixed together to provide variety. The seeds should also be dry and free of moulds; both shelled and unshelled peanuts should be examined for mould. Peanuts are attacked by a mould that produces strong toxins (aflatoxins) that can cause liver damage; fed over a period of time, they can cause the death of a bird.

Soaked seeds (after thorough washing) may be fed to young birds that are having trouble in breaking hard seeds, and to birds during breeding and moulting seasons. The seeds should be soaked in warm water for about 24 hours; this will stimulate the germination of the seeds and germination increase the protein, vitamin content and their availability. Soaked seeds provide an ideal medium for the growth of moulds and fungi. Hence, left over soaked seeds are not to be given next day. The containers are to be cleaned and dried properly.

Birds can also be fed green plant materials such as green leafy vegetables, carrot tops, and spinach in limited amounts. Green material must be thoroughly washed to remove any residue of pesticides or other chemicals.

Birds cannot grind up their food since they don't have teeth. They can break the seeds open with their beaks, but the actual grinding of the feed takes place in the proventriculus or gizzard. This is accomplished with the aid of grit that must be supplied in their diet.

Grit Feeding

Grit is available in two forms, soluble and insoluble. The soluble form is usually oyster shell that breaks down and serves as a source of calcium. The soluble grit also meets the calcium needs for egg shell formation; example cuttlefish. These are marine mollusks and are good sources of calcium. Cuttlefish need to be cut into pieces to facilitate their feeding in case of small birds. The insoluble form is usually the stones and crushed granite, which provides the primary base for which the feed material is rubbed and worked against to grind the feed. Grit should be available to the birds at all times.

Feeding of Cage Birds

Cage birds can be differentiated into various categories based on the feeding behaviour. Munias, parakeets and budgerigar are seed eaters or hard bills.

Table 2. Classification of food consumption patterns of birds*

Category	Examples
1. Generalist feeder: omnivore (polyphage)	Tinamous, bustards, quail, pheasants, cranes, crows
2. Specialist feeder: oligovore (oligophage)	
(i) Animal matter: faunivore (zoophage)	Penguins, grebes, petrels, auks, herons, albatrosses, terns
(a) Invertebrate: microfaunivore Arthropod	Plovers, sandpipers, some ducks
Insect: insectivore	Cuckoos, nightjars, swift, woodpeckers, swallows, wrens, thrushes
Crustacean: crustivore	Crab plovers, some rails, penguins and auks
Mollusk: moluscivore	Limpkins, snail kite, oystercatchers, kiwi
Zooplankton: planktonivore	Flamingos
(b) Vertebrate: macrofaunivore	
Fish: piscivore	Loons, pelicans, storks, cormorants, mergansers, osprey
Terrestrial vertebrates: carnivore	Hawks, owls, eagles, falcons, vultures
(ii) Plant matter: florivore (phytophage)	
(a) Browser:	
Leaves, buds, shoots, grasses: Herbivore	Ostrich, grouse, some ducks
Grasses: graminivore (phoephage)	Geese, swans
Leaves: folivore	Hoatzin
(b) Concentrate selectors	
Grains and hard seeds: granivore	Sparrows, finches, waxbills, some ducks, pigeons and parrots
Fruits: frugivore	Toucans, manikins, birds of paradise, tanagers, some pigeons and bulbuls
Nectar: nectarivore	Hummingbirds, lorikeets, sunbirds, honeyeaters
Fungus: fungivore	Pygmy parrot
Lichens: lichenivore	
Moss: bryophytivore	
Exudates (saps, gums, resins): exudativore	Sapsuckers

* Klasing, K.C. (1998) Comparative Animal Nutrition published by CAB International, Wallingford, Oxon OX10 8DE, UK; Greek (-phage) terms are shown in parentheses and are considered synonymous with the more commonly used Latin (-vore) terms.

Myna is insect eater or soft bill. Koels, pigeons and doves fall into two classes, seed-eaters (granivores) and fruit-eaters (frugivores). Generally insect-eater requires more care in feeding whereas seed-eaters are easily fed.

Feeds include legume seeds, cereal grains, millets and small millets and green leafy vegetables. Minerals and vitamins should also be provided. Soaked seeds are better than unsoaked seeds. Cuttlefish bone and shell grit (soluble grit) should also be made available to seed eating birds as a source of calcium and other minerals. Insoluble grit enables a seed eater to digest its feed properly.

Feeding of hand-reared birds: Hand-reared birds are in great demand because they are usually tamer and more easily handled. Birds that are hand-reared need to be provided a brooder or heating pad so that the birds can be kept warm. A spoon bent up on the sides makes an ideal tool for hand-feeding young birds.

Hand-feeding is very time consuming. Newly hatched birds need to be fed every 3 or 4 hours. Feeding is required from early morning to late evening. Feeds commonly used are dry cereals, fruits, and canned baby food. These foods are mixed with water in a blender and then heated to make it warm. Mineral and vitamin supplements can be added. As the birds get older, they can be gradually weaned from the liquid diet to seeds.

Feeding of Orphan Birds

Nidicolous Chicks and Nidifugous Chicks

Young birds are of two types: Nidicolous chicks (altricial birds) and nidifugous chicks (precocial). Altricial birds require nourishment since they are incapable of moving around on their own soon after hatching or being born. Species whose young are immediately or quickly mobile are known as precocial. Nidicolous chicks (altricial birds) are generally blind, helpless and more or less naked (nestling). They need much personal care, since they hatch at an early stage of development. Nidifugous chicks (precocial) have longer incubation period and they leave the shell clad in down feathers. They have the ability to run about and pick up food for themselves.

Feeding and nutrition: The best feeder is thin tipped spatulate wooden stick or (match stick). This helps to push back the feed on bird's tongue. It is important not to fill the mouth with feed, as this may block the wind pipe and cause suffocation. Young nestling require frequent feeding in every 20-30 minutes. It is generally safe to continue feeding until the bird ceases to gape (open the mouth wide).

Depending upon the type of species, the feed may be boiled mashed egg, biscuit meal, insects, larvae, minced earthworm, bread thoroughly soaked in milk (otherwise the dripped milk may enter the trachea and may cause aspiration). Banana and other soft fruits can also be given.

It is a good policy to do feeding, watering and cleaning at the same time and place each day, if possible by the same person. Birds quickly become accustomed to such routine. One should always remember to move slowly and deliberately around birds and not to make sudden loud sounds as birds are very easily frightened by unaccustomed movements or sounds.

Feeding passerine group of birds: The passerine group of birds are born in a warm nest, either naked or with a covering of down. Song birds are passerines while other birds are non-passerine. They should be housed in their own nest or replica of it with a thick pad of cotton covering them. If possible two or more nestling should be kept together. When the pad is removed, the nestling gape (open the mouth wide) reflexively for food. After feeding, they usually elevate their cloacal regions to the edge of the nest to defecate. The dropping is contained in a thin membrane and should be removed with a teaspoon.

Chicks are fed until they stop gaping. Young birds grow quickly. As growth occurs, feeding intervals are lengthened and large food items given. Once young bird begins to eat without aid, they can be introduced to water. A large stone placed in a shallow dish of water gives the birds some security, prevents spillage and enables them to bathe.

Dried egg based food with cereal and dried insect can be given. It is important to add as much live insect feed as possible. Hardboiled egg and or scraped raw liver in small quantities can be given if no dried food is available. When the birds grow older, the diet should be more closely approximate the adult diet (e.g. more cereal for seed-eating birds)

Parrots and pigeons: Parrots and pigeons initially feed their naked young on a regurgitated crop secretion (crop milk). It is possible to rear chick from a tender age by imitating the parents, using a small syringe containing a quantity of milk-based baby food.

Young birds should be placed in a small cardboard box and bedded on wood shaving within a cage kept at about 90° F (32.2° C) for the first 4 or 5 days. The amount of food to be given varies with the species.

Generally 1 ml will do for a bird of pigeon size, offered every 3 hours during the day. The degree of crop distension indicates the amount of food required. Care should be taken, as overfilling of crop can lead to disease.

Common Diet for Different Category of Pet Birds

Seed-eaters: Largest and most popular cage and aviary birds are seed eaters. These birds live mainly on seeds, but also eat fruit, insects, egg and green food. Fruit and green feed contain a lot of important nutrients, but too much of these will give rise to problem such as diarrhoea.

Green feed is good during breeding season. During breeding season, seed eaters should be introduced with insects and worms so that they will recognize the feed and feed their young with insects and worms.

Animal protein food has proven to be very valuable especially in the period leading up to the breeding time as well as during and after the breeding time too.

The bird's main diet should consist of its seed mix supplemented with some green grasses/leaves, insects, and egg to avoid deficiency.

Diets for finches (kind of small birds) and caneries: Diet includes cereal grains, millets, and sunflower seed. A good mineralized grit (shell grit / cuttlebone) should always be available. Many finches required animal protein in their diets, especially to the young ones. Finches enjoy green grasses, such as those found in the garden.

Parrots and cockatoos: Most are basically seed eaters, but one group, the lories and lorikeets feed predominately on nectar, pollen and fruit.

Small parrots (Budgerigar or Red rumped parrots): Diet includes cereal grains, millets, and legume seed. A good mineralized grit (shell grit / cuttlebone) should always be available.

Medium parrots (cockatiel): Diet includes cereal grains, millets, legume seed and sunflower seed. Green feed, fruit (apple, pear, orange) are also to be fed. A good mineralized grit (shell grit / cuttlebone) should always be available. Many birds enjoy chewing on the leaves and bark of native trees.

Larger parrots (cockatoos, macaws and African grey parrot): Diet includes cereal grains, millets, legume seed, groundnut seed and sunflower seed along with grit and shell grit. It is essential that these species have a wide variety of fruit (apple, orange/mango, guava, chilly fruit, tomato), vegetables (green banana, cucumber, carrot), bread and green branches of non-poisonous tree. Feather problem are common in larger parrots, as they are prone to boredom; this situation can be partially alleviated by adding something to chew on.

Baby cockatoos and baby parrots: For baby cockatoos and baby parrots, the feed is prepared as follows. Mix the dry ingredients: ½ cup baby food cereal, 1/8 teaspoon salt and ½ teaspoon fine cuttle fish bone meal; add 1 teaspoon corn syrup or honey, 2 fresh egg yolks and then milk or water to make a soup like mixture. Boil over low heat 3-5 minutes, stirring gently. Cool it to add 4 drops vitamins supplement. Feed the mixture with a spoon.

The baby birds should be fed three to six times daily. The crop is usually visible as semitransparent bag at the base of the neck so it is possible to determine the amount of food left after the last feeding.

Lories and lorikeets: Lories and lorikeets feed on nectar and pollen. Nectar foods are usually powders that need to be mixed with water and provided to the birds in special feeders. Lories and lorikeets also eat fruit.

The feed may be prepared as follows. One cup baby cereal food is mixed with one cup of warm water, two table spoon condensed milk, two table spoon honey, raw sugar or glucose and six drops of liquid vitamins (used for human babies). The feed should be changed twice daily.

In a separate pan offer mixed fruit, apple, pear, grapes, papaya, soaked raisins, tomato etc. Offer cereal grains, millets, sunflower seed. These species also like to chew on bark, leaves and blossoms of most of the trees.

Pigeons and doves: The majority of the species are seed eaters. They require variety of seeds of appropriate size (cereal grains, millets, legume seeds) and a good mineralized grit. Grit is especially important, because pigeons swallow their food whole and grind it in the gizzard. A good mineralized grit (shell grit / cuttlebone) should always be available.

Mynah birds: Mynah birds will not eat seeds and do not need grit or cuttlefish in their diet. Mynah birds are fed special soft bill pellets. Mynah birds also need fruit in their diet, apple slices, grapes, orange slices, and banana slices are the most common. Dried fruits can also be used, provided they are soaked and rinsed off before feeding.

Mynah birds also like live food such as meal worms. Mynahs, particularly when they are breeding, like live food, like flies, spiders, moths, snails, butterflies, crickets, beatles, etc. Instead of live food we can use a combination of minced raw lean meat and equal parts of poultry crumbs and fine puppy meal which have been soaked with hot water until soft. We can also provide hardboiled egg made into mash. Also add sweet ripe fruits in the diet.

Feeding Schedules of Pet Birds*

Name of the bird	Diet prescribed	Quantity per day	Additional supplements**
Love birds	Apple	30 g	
	Banana	30 g	
	Thinai/small millets	10.0 g	
	Paddy / Mixed Grains**	10 g	
	White Bengal Gram	05 g	
	Onion	10 g	
	Green gram	10 g	
	Greens	10 g	
	Shell grit	04 g	
Small parrot: Budgerigar	*Thinai or korralu* or small millets	10 g	
	Green gram	05 g	
	Bengal gram	05 g	
	Coriander leaves, palak, onion	10 g	
	Shell grit	10 g	
Medium parrot: Cockatile	Green gram	10 g	
	Mixed grains**	10 g	
	Thinai / small millets	10 g	
	Bengal gram	10 g	
	Greens	10 g	
	Onion	10 g	
	Shell grit	04 g	
Koel/ Large parrot: Cockatoo	Mixed grains**	50 g	
	Apple	75 g/variable size	
	Sathukudi/orange / mango	50 g /variable size	
	Guava	100 g /variable size	
	Chilly fruit	05 g	
	Tomato	50g	
	Groundnut without shell	50 g	

	Tapioca / sweet potato	50 g	
	Bread slice	1no	
	Egg boiled	1 no	
	Green banana	75 g	
	Sunflower seeds	10 g	
	Carrot	50 g	
Large parrot: Macaw	Bread slice	01 no	
	Green banana	140 g /variable size	
	Bengal gram	25 g	
	Apple	75 g /variable size	
	Orange / mango	75 g /variable size	
	Guava	100 g /variable size	
	Groundnut without shell	50 g	
	Chilly fruit	25 g	
	Garlic	10 g	
	Cucumber	50 g	
	Greens	20 g	
	Shell grit	20 g	
Macaw, Cockatoo	Sri Venkateswara Zoological Park, Tirupati follow	Honey 10g, groundnut seeds 30g, mixed grains and seeds (paddy, sunflower seeds and kusum seeds 5+20 +5) 30g and fruit mix (banana, apples, sweetlime, grapes, guava/mango, Bengal gram) 100g are given in the forenoon.	Fruit mix (banana, apples, sweetlime, grapes, guava/mango, Bengal gram) 100g are given in the afternoon.
Rainbow lory	Sri Venkateswara Zoological Park, Tirupati follow	Bread 10g, milk 20ml, honey 10g, fruit mix 50g and mixed grains and seeds (paddy, sunflower seeds	

		and kusum seeds 5+20+5) 30g are given in the forenoon per day	
Pigeon (Columbidae) (Schedule IV)	Mixed grains** White Bengal gram Green gram Shell grit	25 g 20 g 25 g 20 g	
Dove (Columbidae) (Schedule IV)	Bread slice Mixed grains** White Bengal gram Shell grit	1 no 25 g 20 g 01 g	
Peafowl (*Pavo cristatus*) (Schedule I, Part III)	Cabbage Mixed grains** Paddy White Bengal gram Greens Garlic Groundnut without shell Green gram Onion Shell grit	25 g 25 g 25 g 50 g 100 g 10 g 50 g 25 g 25 g 20 g	
Peacock, pheasant (*Polyplectron bicalcaratum*) (Schedule I, Part III), jungle fowl (Phasianidae) (Schedule IV)	Sri Venkateswara Zoological Park, Tirupati follow	Poultry feed (layer) 120g and a few meal worms are given in the forenoon.	Palak / green leaves 50g and onion 25 g are given in the afternoon.
Mynah (*Sturnidae*) (Schedule IV)	Mixed grains** Bread slice Greens Onion Assorted fruits Shell grit	50 g 1 no 25 g 25 g 10 g 02 g	

* Adapted from diet sheet during 2011-2012, Arignar Anna Zoological Park, Vandalur, Chennai-48.

** Composition of mixed grains: paddy, 20%; sorghum, 20%; cumbu, 20%; ragi, 20% and wheat 20%; Tuesday is fasting for all animals except pregnant animals, ailing animals, nursing animals, aquatic birds and other special cases

Feeding Schedules of Birds*

Name of the bird	Diet prescribed	Quantity per day	Additional supplements**
House sparrow (*Picchuka in telugu*)	Paddy, bajra, ragi	15 g	
Ducks (Anatidae) (Schedule IV)	Paddy	100 g	
Bengal goose (Anatidae; Schedule IV)	Wheat bran White Bengal gram Carrot Cabbage	50 g 25 g 25 g 25 g	
Flamingo (*Phoenicopteridae*) (Schedule IV)	Thinai Wheat bran Mixed grains#	150 g 50 g 50 g	
Black swan (*Anatidae*) (Schedule IV)	Cabbage Wheat Paddy Cucumber White Bengal gram Bread slice Carrot Shell grit	25 g 50 g 50 g 100 g 25 g 1 No 25 g 5 g	
Brahmini kite/ Pariah kite	Beef with bone Or rat	500 g 2 Nos weekly once	Chick 2 Nos weekly once Fish 200 g weekly once
Bengal vulture (*Accipitridae*) (Schedule IV)	Beef with bone Or rat	1 kg 2 Nos weekly once	Chick 5 Nos weekly once Fish 500 g weekly once
Owl Barn owl	Beef with bone	250 g	

(*Tytoninae*) (Schedule IV)	Or rat	150 g 2 Nos per day	Chicks 10 g weekly once
Horn owl	Rat 100 to 150 g Or chicks	2 Nos 2 Nos weekly once	
Stork (Painted stork Sarus crane) (Ciconiidae) (Schedule IV)	Fish	500 g	
Heron (Ardeidae) and Egret (pond heron, purple heron, night heron, grey heron; cattle egret (Schedule IV)	Fish	200–500 g	
Pelican (Spot billed and rosy) (Pelicanidae; Schedule IV)	Fish	0.75 kg - 1 kg	
Shikra	Chopped beef	150 g	Rat of 100 to 150 g 2 Nos (weekly twice)

* Adapted from diet sheet during 2011-2012, Arignar Anna Zoological Park, Vandalur, Chennai-48.
** Only iodised salt is provided for salt supplementation. Tuesday is fasting for all animals except pregnant animals, ailing animals, nursing animals, aquatic birds and other special cases.
# Composition of mixed grains: paddy, 20%; sorghum, 20%; cumbu, 20%; ragi, 20% and wheat 20%

Precautions to be taken while Feeding Fish

Otters, badgers, pelicans, penguins, gharials, dolphins, ferrets, pole cats, mink etc. are often fed with fish.

Gill regions in the fish need to be examined for the freshness. Rotten fish or fish with more pungent smell are to be avoided.

Avoid the feeding of fish like carps and herring that contain the enzyme 'thiaminase' since this may destroy the thiamine in the diet.

Cooked fish or fish like butter fish and mackerel may be used. Usage of oily fish like herring may lead to the oxidation of vitamin A and E in the diet.

Walk-in-aviary and Open Bird Park

Arignar Anna Zoological Park in Vandalur has a Walk-in-aviary which housed migratory birds. The visitors of the zoo can enjoy the sight of these birds. It is planning to set up a 'open bird park' on a two-hectare plot adjacent to the 'sambar safari'. The open park will have nectar-bearing flowering plants and a specially-created small pond with fish. Nest boxes on tree branches (along with food trays), sand and ash bath on the ground are provided. Dung, farmyard manure, leaf litter and fallen branches have been strewn about so that insects and worms can breed there. The presence of insects and worms will attract he insectivorous-birds.

The 'open bird park' is expected to attract fruit-eating birds, insect-eating birds and grain-eating birds; all nearly 30 species of free-ranging terrestrial birds - red-vented bulbul, red-whiskered bulbul, babblers, coppersmith barbet, grey francolin, wood shrike, Indian robin and hoopoe, etcetera migratory birds will arrive.

19

Metabolic Diseases in Birds

Metabolic Disorders

Metabolic disorders in caged birds may be due to deficiency of one or many indispensable elements; imbalance of calcium and phosphorus may cause bone disorder; excess caloric intake may cause obesity, fat deposits and fatty liver.

Metabolic Bone Disease in Captive Aviary Species

Rickets is encountered in growing birds especially in birds which have long or large legs and is caused by calcium and phosphorus imbalance and deficiency of vitamin D. But osteomalacia is a disease of adult birds and causes are same.

The affected birds show weakness, anorexia, polydipsia, intermittent loose droppings. Poor feather growth and chewing at plumage are observed in such birds. Upper and lower beaks may not oppose each other properly and prehension of food is faulty. Hunch backed appearance, improper calcification of eggs (eggs become softer) and retention of eggs without laying (due to lack of calcium) are also observed.

The clinical signs include the bones become thin, soft, painful and fragile and can break spontaneously when a bird is handled. Affected bird may appear drowsy, feather picked and reluctant to perch, move or fly. The female lay brittle eggs or egg production may cease.

Treatment includes calcium and vitamin D supplements. For calcium, calcium gluconate or lactate can be given orally. For vitamin D - cod-liver oil can be placed on seed, to drinking water or by subcutaneous injection. Improvement of the diet by adding oyster shell grit, fish and cooked vegetables is also to be followed simultaneously.

Other Calcium Related Metabolic Derangements

Egg binding: Egg binding is commonly encountered in many aviary species. Along with other causes, calcium deficiency due to multiple metabolic derangements plays a significant role. Hence, in egg bound aviary species, calcium borogluconate is given by intravenous or subcutaneous route and this helps in the improvement of the tonicity of the musculatures and helps in the rapid expulsion of egg.

Malformed eggs: Malformed egg especially shell-less egg or partially shelled egg or soft-shelled egg may be laid by multiple aviary species reared under captive conditions. In addition to the salpingitis, the etiological factor for this might be the existence of imbalance in calcium and phosphorus levels.

An **imbalance** in calcium, phosphorus and vitamin D is commonly encountered **in parrots** and the problem arises as a result of their customary diet of high oil-bearing foods such as sunflower seeds and peanuts. This, in addition to the metabolic derangements, produce a variety of clinical expressions in the affected wild birds reared in captivity.

Hypothyroidism in Captive Aviary Species

A deficiency of iodine in the diet can result in decreased secretion of hormone thyroxin. There may be hypertrophy of thyroid gland resulting in goiter. The affected birds will reveal change of voice i.e. a respiratory noise heard as a characteristic 'click' and this is due to the pressure of the enlarged thyroid on syrinx and the lower trachea. In addition to the obesity and dullness, there may be ruffled feathers in the affected bird. The affected birds are unable to maintain body temperature when exposed to environmental change. Birds have increased blood cholesterol.

Gout

This condition is more common in captive birds. Especially hawks, eagles, kites, vultures, falcons are highly susceptible in addition to ostrich, cassowary, peafowls, budgerigars, love birds, parakeets, goose, duck, etc.

Gout may be true gout (deposition of monosodium urate crystals) or pseudo gout (deposition of any crystal other than sodium urate). It may be visceral gout and articular gout or synovial gout. Visceral gout is deposition of whitish urate or uric acid crystals as white coloured powder or foci often on mainly epicardium and liver and also on kidney and on peritoneum. Localization of urate crystals may vary from individual to individual.

Synovial gout is deposition of urate crystals in and around the joints. Small white nodules called as tophi or tophus is clearly visible to the unaided eyes. The possible causes include renal problems, nutritional and stress. Renal problems (infection / inflammation / renal lesions due to nephrotoxic substances like gentamicin and anti-inflammatory drugs like salicylates, probenecids, phenylbutazone etc.) are the basic cause because liver and renal tissues are involved in production of urate crystals.

Nutritional causes may include increased protein intake without provision of water. Stress leading to dehydration or dehydration due to diseases that lead ultimately reduced renal blood flow and ultimately gout occurs.

See Appendix for information on Avian atherosclerosis.

References

Arora, B.M. 2001.Dietary Husbandry of Wild Mammals. AIZWV and Central Zoo Authority, New Delhi, India.

AVMA. 2008. One Health: A New Professional Imperative: AVMA One Health Initiative Task Force Report; Available from: http://www.qvmq.org/KB/Resources/Reports/Documents/onehealth_final.pdf

Billinis, C. 2013 Wildlife diseases that pose a risk to small ruminants and their farmers. Small Ruminant Research, 110, 2-3, 67-70.

Carta, T., Alvarez, J., J.M.Perez de la Lastra and C.Gortazar (2013) Wildlife and paratuberculosis: A review. Research in Veterinary Science, 94, 191-197.

Das, A., Katole, S., Choubey, M. Gupta, S.P., Saini, M., Kumar, V. and Swarup, D. 2013. Feed consumption, diet digestibility and mineral utilization in captive blackbuck (Antelope cervicapra) fed different levels of concentrates. Journal of Animal Physiology and Animal Nutrition, 97, 1, 80-90.

Das, A., M.Saini, Shrikant Katole, A.S.Kullu and A.K.Sharma (2012). Effect of feeding different levels of wheat-roti on nutrient utilization and blood metabolite profile in semi-captive Asiatic elephants (Elephas maximus), page 120; IN: Pattanaik, A.K., Dutta, N., Verma, A.K., Jadhav, S.E., Dhuria, R.K. and Chaudhary, L.C. (Eds). 2012. Animal Nutrition Research Strategies for Food Security: Abstracts. Proceedings of 8th Biennial Animal Nutrition Association Conference, November 28-30, 2012, Bikaner, India, 256 pp

Das, A., Saini, M. and Swarup, D. (2012). Feeding and Nutrition of Wild Animals in Captivity pp 305-328 IN: [Editors: Dr U.R.Mehra (Chief Editor), Putan Singh and A.K.Verma] "Animal Nutrition Advances &

Developments" published by Satish Serial Publishing House, Delhi-110033 ISBN 81-89304-89-5; xiv plus 810 pages]

Depauw, S., Hesta, M.,Whitehouse-Tedd, K., Vanhaecke, L., Verbrugghe, A. and Janssens, G.P.J. 2013. Animal fibre: The forgotten nutrient in strict carnivores? First insights in the cheetah. Journal of Animal Physiology and Animal Nutrition, 97, 1, 146-154.

Diet sheet during 2011-2012, Arignar Anna Zoological Park, Vandalur, Chennai-48.

Ehrlich, Paul (1988). *The Birder's Handbook*. New York: Simon & Schuster. ISBN 0-671-65989-8.

E-learning courses - VMD 512 at Tanuvas and National Agricultural Innovation Project on "Development of E-Courses For B.V.Sc. & A.H. Degree Programme"

Hasselquist, D and Nilsson, Jan-Åke (2009). Maternal transfer of antibodies in vertebrates: trans-generational effects on offspring immunity. Phil. Trans. R. Soc. B 12 January 2009, 364 (1513) 51-60.

Jacob.V.Cheeran, 2004 Textbook of Wild & Zoo Animals Care and Management.

Karma, D.N., Neeta Agarwal, Chaudhary, L.C., Pathak, N.N., Garg, A.K. and Sastry, V.R.B. (eds) 1999. Nutrition and Feeding of Wild Mammals - A short course from Dec 23, 1999 to Jan 21, 2000; Centre of Advanced Studies in Animal Nutrition, Izatnagar - 243122.

Klasing, K.C. (1998) Comparative Animal Nutrition published by CAB International, Wallingford, Oxon OX10 8DE, UK

Monath TP. Vaccines against diseases transmitted from animals to humans: A one health paradigm. Vaccine (2013), http://dx.doi.org/10.1016/j.vaccine.2013.09.029

Nagy, K.A. 2005. Review: Field metabolic rate and body size The Journal of Experimental Biology 208, 1621-1625

Nofs, S.A., Atmar, R.L., Keitel, W.A., Hanlon, C., Stanton, J.J., Tan, J, Flanagan, J.P., Howard, L and Ling, P.D. 2013. Prenatal passive transfer of maternal immunity in Asian elephants (*Elephas maximus*). Veterinary Immunology and Immunopathology, 153: 308-311.

Pattanaik, A.K. (2012). Nutrition and Feeding of Pet Animals pp 221-258 IN: [Editors: Dr U.R.Mehra (Chief Editor), Putan Singh and A.K.Verma] "Animal Nutrition Advances & Developments" published by Satish Serial Publishing House, Delhi-110033 ISBN 81-89304-89-5; xiv plus 810 pages]

Prasad, D.A., D.V.Reddy and A.S.N.Murthy (1983). Evaluation of complete rations (Conventional/ unconventional ingredients) and prediction of body composition of lambs from tritiated water space and bodyweight Journal of Nuclear Agriculture and Biology 12: 29-32.

Reddy, D.V. (1981) M.V.Sc thesis "Effect of protein - energy relationships on performance and prediction of body composition of Large White Yorkshire pigs" submitted to Andhra Pradesh Agricultural University, Hyderabad.

Robins, C.T. (1993). Wildlife Feeding and Nutrition, Academic Press, Inc.

Sanyal, R.H. (1892). A handbook of the management of wild animals in captivity in Lower Bengal, Bengal Secretariat Press, Calcutta. Cited by Das, A., Saini, M. and Swarup, D. (2012)

Sorensen, A., van Beest, F.M. and Brook, R.K. (2013) Impacts of wildlife baiting and supplemental feeding on infectious disease transmission risk: a synthesis of knowledge, Preventive Veterinary Medicine http:// dx.doi.org/10.1016/j.prevetmed.2013.11.010

Shrikant Katole, A.Das, M.Saini and A.K.Sharma (2012) Nutrient utilization in semi-captive Asiatic elephants (*Elephas maximus*) fed different types of supplements, page 96; IN: Pattanaik, A.K., Dutta, N., Verma, A.K., Jadhav, S.E., Dhuria, R.K. and Chaudhary, L.C. (Eds). 2012. Animal Nutrition Research Strategies for Food Security: Abstracts. Proceedings of 8th Biennial Animal Nutrition Association Conference, November 28-30, 2012, Bikaner, India, 256 pp

Sreekumar, D., R.Sreekrishnan, R.S.Rajkumar and K.Afsal (2011) Preliminary report on the bird diversity in the Veterinary College Campus, Puducherry. ZOO'S Print, volume XXVI, Numer 10, October 2011.

Starck, J. (1998). *Avian Growth and Development.* Oxford Oxfordshire: Oxford University Press. ISBN 0-19-510608-3.

"The Wildlife (Protection) Act, 1972 with the Wildlife (Protection) Amendment Act, 2002" PDF 148 pages Downloaded from internet - The Gazette of India Published by Government of India, January 20, 2003.

Van Soest, P.J. (1981). "Nutritional Ecology of the Ruminant" O. and B. Books, Corvallis, Oregan, USA.

Van Soest, P.J., E.S.Dierenfeld and N.L.Conklin (1995) Digestive strategies and limitations of ruminants pp 581-600 **IN:** *W.v.Engelhardt et al (eds) Ruminant Physiology: Digestion, Metabolism, Growth and Reproduction, Proceedings of the Eighth International Symposium on Ruminant Physiology*

Verkest, K.R. (2013) Is the metabolic syndrome a useful clinical concept in dogs? A review of the evidence. The Veterinary Journal, http://dx.doi.org/10.1016/j.tvjl.2013.09.057

Appendix

1. Altricial and Precocial Birds or Mammals

Altricial: Species whose young are incapable of moving around on their own soon after hatching or being born are referred to altricial. Altricial, meaning "requiring nourishment", refers to a pattern of growth and development in such organisms. Hence altricial refers to the need for young to be fed and taken care of for a long duration (Ehrlich, Paul, 1988). Altricial young are born helpless (closed eyes are common) and require care for a specific amount of time. Among mammals, marsupials and most rodents are altricial. Cats, dogs, and humans are some of the best-known altricial organisms.

Altricial birds are less able to contribute nutrients in the pre-natal stage; their eggs are smaller and their young still in need of much attention and protection from predators. Altricial birds include passerines, cape vulture, double-crested cormorant, herons, hawks, woodpeckers, owls. Semi-altricial and semi-precocial birds include auks, petrels and terns.

Precocial: Species whose young are immediately or quickly mobile are known as precocial. In precocial animals the young have open eyes, have hair or down, have large brains, and are immediately mobile and somewhat able to flee from, or defend themselves against, predators. For example, with ground-nesting birds such as chicks, ducks or turkeys, the young are ready to leave the nest in one or two days. Among mammals, most ungulates are precocial, being able to walk almost immediately after birth.

Precocial birds are able to provide protein-rich eggs and thus their young hatch in the fledgling stage - able to protect themselves from predators (chicks, ducks or turkeys) and the females have less post-natal involvement. Some more precocial birds include waterfowl and quail.

"Altricial" and "precocial" refer to developmental stage, while **"nidifugous"** and **"nidicolous"** refer to leaving or staying at the nest (Starck, J. 1998).

The two strategies result in different brain sizes of the newborns compared to adults. Precocial animals' brains are large at birth relative to their body size. Hence, they have ability to fend for themselves. However, as adults, their brains are not much bigger or more able. Altricial animals' brains are relatively small at birth (but their brains continue to grow), thus they need care and protection at young stage. As adults, altricial animals end up with comparatively larger brains than their precocial counterparts. Thus the altricial species have a wider skill set at maturity (Ehrlich, Paul, 1988).

2. Passerine birds: The most prominent characteristic of passerine birds is the anisodactyl arrangement of toes. These birds have four toes, three facing forward and one backward, which allows the bird to easily cling to both horizontal and nearly vertical perches, including branches and tree trunks. These birds also have an adaptation in their legs that gives them extra strength for perching, so the birds are able to perch easily even when sleeping.

Passerine are birds, like house sparrow (*Passer domesticus*). In addition to the toes, there is a distinction by the birds voice boxes (their 'syrinyxes'). There are a number of birds that have a passerine foothold, but a more primitive syrinx than the true songbirds. About 60 percent of all bird species are passerines. Songbirds are passerines, others are not.

Non-passerine foothold: Budgerigar bird has two toes forward and two backward.

3. Some Wild Animals

Gaur or Indian bison (Bos gaurus): Gaurs are seen in Central India-Madhya Pradesh and Chhatisghar, Western Ghats southwards from south Maharashtra, Mudumalai Anaimalai, Dindigul region and Palani regions. This is wild bovidae and considered to be one of the ancestors of the mithun. Mithun and gaur have been adopted on the diet of domestic cattle.

Nilgiri Tahr (*Hemitragus hylocrius*): Seen in Nilgiris to Anaimalais and southwards along the Western ghats from 4000-6000 feet. Population census was recorded by direct sighting and by indirect sighting through identification of the faecal pellets and pug marks of the animals in high altitude areas ranging between 3500 feet and 6000 feet above the mean sea level. Global Positional System has been used for temporal and special mapping of the entire Tahr habitat.

Nilgai: The male nilgai (*Boselaphus tragocamelus*) is also called as 'blue bull'. They are seen in Himalayas to Mysore (Not seen in Bengal, Assam, Malabar Coast and Tamil Nadu). These are generally seen in dry deciduous and thorn forests of Indian peninsula and are large horse like animals.

Kangaroo: A kangaroo is a marsupial mammal. It is a macropod which means 'big foot'. A kangaroo moves by hopping on its powerful hind legs. It can also leap over obstacles up to 10 feet high.

Porpoise: Porpoise is a sea animal rather like a dophin or small whale. Sea animals include walrus, conger-eel, seal, dophin, whale, shark, starfish, swordfish, dogfish, jellfish.

Species with many young: Laboratory rat, guinea pig, brown hare, mink, striped skunk, domestic rabbit, domestic dog, domestic pig, and American black bear;

Ungulates with single offspring: Black-tailed deer, domestic sheep, red deer, reindeer, elk, domestic cow, domestic horse, caribou, muskox, mule deer, mountain goat, Dorcas gazelle, and ibex;

Ungulates with twins: Black-tailed deer, mule deer, and domestic sheep

Primates: human and baboon

Marsupial: tammar wallaby

Caecotrophs are the soft materials that are often consumed directly from the anal region. Animals like rabbits and hares produce these soft faecal pellets that have high protein, and water contents with increased amounts of vitamin B complex.

4. Table 1. Composition (%) and Energy content (kcal/g) of mammalian milks for eutherians at mid-lactation and for marsupials (embryonic marsupial confined to the pouch and after vacating the pouch)*

Group or species	Water	Fat	Protein	Sugar	Ash	Energy
Marsupials						
Eastern quoll						
0-9 weeks	83.0	4.5	5.8	5.8	-	0.96
10-22 weeks	68.5	14.2	8.0	4.8	-	1.94
Potoroo						
0-15 weeks	76.0	2.0	6.5	11.0	-	0.84
16-25 weeks	67.5	13.5	12.0	3.5	-	1.73

Red-necked wallaby						
0-33 weeks	80.0	5.0	5.0	9.5	-	0.73
34-57 weeks	73.7	13.2	7.3	3.2	-	1.63
Tammar wallaby						
0-20 weeks	82.0	4.0	4.3	8.0	-	0.93
21-45 weeks	70.0	16.0	10.0	3.0	-	2.14
Tasmanian bettong						
0-18 weeks	76.0	2.0	3.5	10.0	-	0.83
19-24 weeks	65.0	15.0	7.5	2.0	-	1.79
Insectivores						
White-toothed shrew	48.8	31.9	9.7	-	2.6	-
Primates						
Baboons	86.0	4.6	1.5	7.7	0.3	0.80
Human	87.6	4.1	0.8	6.8	0.2	0.69
Lemurs	-	2.3	1.9	6.7	0.3	0.58
Talapoin monkey	87.7	3.0	2.1	7.2	0.3	0.67
Lagomorphs						
Domestic rabbit	68.8	15.2	10.3	1.8	1.8	2.04
Easterncottontail rabbit	64.8	14.4	15.8	2.7	2.1	2.33
European brown hare	67.8	14.8	10.3	1.6	-	2.00
Rodents						
Brown rat	77.9	8.8	8.1	3.8	1.2	1.43
Chinchilla	-	11.2	7.3	1.7	1.0	1.50
European beaver	65.9	19.0	11.2	1.7	1.1	2.46
Golden hamster	77.4	4.9	9.4	4.9	1.4	1.20
Guinea pig	82.5	5.7	6.3	4.8	0.8	1.08
House mouse	70.7	13.1	9.0	3.0	1.5	1.85
Carnivores-Fissipeds						
Arctic fox	71.4	13.5	11.1	3.0	1.0	1.98
Brown bear	66.4	18.5	8.5	2.3	1.5	2.28
Domestic cat	-	10.8	10.6	3.7	1.0	1.74
Domestic dog	77.3	9.5	7.5	3.8	1.1	1.46
Mink	78.3	7.3	5.6	4.5	1.0	1.18
Racoon dog	81.4	3.4	7.8	-	1.1	-
Red fox	81.9	5.8	6.7	4.6	0.9	1.09
Striped skunk	69.4	13.8	9.9	3.0	-	1.97
Carnivores-Pinnipeds						
California seal-lion	59.0	30.7	8.6	0.3	-	3.30
Harp seal	48.3	42.2	8.7	0.1	0.7	4.34

Hooded seal	30.3	61.0	4.7	1.0	-	5.88
Northern elephant seal	35.6	48.8	7.6	0.3	-	4.88
Northern fur seal	39.0	49.4	10.2	0.1	0.5	5.09
Southern elephant seal	51.2	39.0	9.0	-	-	4.07
Weddell seal	42.8	42.1	15.8	1.0	-	4.08
Proboscideans						
African elephant	82.7	5.0	4.0	5.3	0.7	0.88
Asian elephant	82.3	7.3	4.5	5.2	0.6	1.12
Perissodactyls						
Ass	91.5	0.6	1.4	6.1	0.4	0.38
Black rhinoceros	91.2	0.2	1.4	6.6	0.3	0.35
Horse	89.5	1.3	1.9	6.9	0.4	0.51
Artiodactyls						
Bactrian camel	84.8	4.3	4.3	-	0.9	-
Black-tailed deer	-	12.6	7.2	4.8	1.4	1.76
Dall sheep	77.1	9.5	7.2	5.3	0.9	1.48
Domestic cow	87.6	3.7	3.2	4.6	0.7	0.71
Domestic pig	79.9	8.3	5.6	5.0	0.9	1.24
Domestic goat	88.0	3.8	2.9	4.7	0.8	0.69
Domestic sheep	81.8	7.3	4.1	5.0	0.8	1.11
Dorcas gazelle	75.9	8.8	8.8	5.7	1.1	1.53
Eland	78.1	9.9	6.3	4.4	1.1	1.43
Gayal	80.0	7.0	6.3	5.2	-	1.20
Giraffe	85.5	4.8	4.0	4.9	0.8	0.86
Ibex	76.7	12.4	5.7	4.4	1.2	1.62
Moose	78.5	10.0	8.4	3.0	1.5	1.51
North American elk	81.0	6.7	5.7	4.2	1.3	1.10
Red deer	78.9	8.5	7.1	4.5	1.4	1.37
Reindeer	73.7	10.9	9.5	3.4	1.3	1.66
Rocky mountain goat	78.7	8.1	6.4	4.3	0.9	1.27
Tahr	-	7.9	5.4	3.1	-	1.14
Water buffalo	83.2	6.5	4.3	4.9	0.8	1.02
White-tailed deer	77.5	7.7	8.2	4.6	1.5	1.35

* Source: Robins, C.T. (1993). Wildlife Feeding and Nutrition, Academic Press, Inc. pp 204-206.

5. Addison's disease (Adrenal cortex insufficiency) or hypoadrenocorticism

The first case of Addison's disease in dogs was recorded in 1953, over 100 years after it was described in humans by Thomas Addison. Adrenal glands do not produce sufficient steroid hormones (glucocorticoids and often mineralocorticoids). Most dogs with Addison's disease will need to be medicated for their entire lives. Medication is of two forms, one to keep their blood potassium and sodium levels (blood electrolytes) optimal and another to replace the cortisol that they can no longer produce. Most of the medications used in the therapy of hypoadrenocorticism cause excessive thirst and urination. It is absolutely vital to provide fresh drinking water for a canine suffering from this disorder.

Addison's disease is not a common disease in pets or humans. Its mirror image, Cushing's disease is much more common.

6. Cushing's disease or hyperadrenocorticism

It is reported that 15% incidence in dogs is due to a tumour in one or both of the adrenal glands, while 85% are due to a benign tumour in pituitary gland (The pituitary gland, 'the master gland' also regulates the function of other endocrine glands in the body). With Cushing's disease, the over-secretion of cortisol triggers so many changes in the dogs' body. Cortisol in excess causes so much damage even to the point of altering the appearance and behaviour of the canine. Cortisol in excess causes polydipsia, polyphagia, polyuria, excessive panting, excessive shedding of hair, etc.

Commercial dog food contains grains, oilseed cakes, animal protein supplements, minerals, vitamins, synthetic ingredients and preservatives, which may in fact trigger allergies and intestinal irritations and thus in turn, making the animal to secrete cortisol all the more. Cortisol is a hormone secreted in response to stress, immune system problems and even when blood glucose levels become imbalanced. Hence better to prepare a bland diet using natural feed ingredients without much processing.

Choose low-purine meat sources such as poultry, rabbit and lamb and eggs. Include fresh fruits and vegetables that provide fibre, antioxidants and electrolytes. Vegetables such as potatoes with the skin, beans, carrots, peas and broccoli are great, while fruits such as apples or other high antioxidant content fruits can also be given in proper amounts in order to provide nutrition and support in treating Cushing's disease. A canine that is suffering from disease can have diminished nutrient absorption. Opting for readily absorbed nutrients from natural food items is necessary. Prepare a high-protein diet; avoid high carbohydrate foods such as cooked brown rice, oats or vegetables such as sweet potatoes, high sodium food items, and food items that have preservatives such as ethoxyquin, propyl gallate, BHA or BHT.

7. Celiac disease or coeliac disease in canines

Canines (cats and dogs) can have celiac disease which is an allergy to a protein called gluten. Gluten proteins are high in proline and glutamine content, which are responsible for poor gluten digestibility. Some of the high molecular weight peptides that are generated in the gastrointestinal tract are involved in an autoimmune enteropathy called celiac disease. Gluten-free diet is the remedy.

Irish Setters are the only breed of dogs known have to true celiac disease (Batt et al., 1984), but many dogs are sensitive to glutenous grains. Untreated celiac disease can lead to malnutrition and damage to the digestive tract. Dogs with celiac disease cannot tolerate gluten, a protein present in wheat, barley and rye. Eating those grains causes an abnormal immune response reaction against gluten that attacks villi small, finger-like projections of the small intestine. If villi are damaged or destroyed (atrophied) the absorption of nutrients from intestinal lumen into bloodstream is disrupted. Hence the affected dogs can become malnourished.

Dogs with celiac disease suffer from diarrheoa or constipation, weakness, vomiting, weight loss and anaemia. A dog with diarrheoa might have stools containing a lot of mucus, an indication that its digestive tract is irritated. Celiac disease can lead to skin problems, including hair loss, itching and flaking, dry skin. Secondary skin infections and chronic ear infections are also observed. The lesions usually show up on the dog's feet, head, neck, ears and stomach.

Irish Setters are the only dogs that have been identified as suffering from true celiac disease. The disease usually shows up in puppies between 4 and 7 months old. The puppies do not gain weight and suffer from chronic diarrheoa. The disease is inherited, passed on from parents to offspring.

A blood test and a biopsy of the small intestine helps veterinarians diagnose celiac disease. Recognizing celiac disease can be difficult because the symptoms mimic those of several other illnesses, including irritable bowel syndrome, parasites and pancreatitis. The symptoms might also be linked to food allergies or sensitivity to gluten, rather than true celiac disease.

Provide wheat- and gluten-free dog foods and treats to the affected dogs.

Batt, R.M., Carter, M.W. and McLean, L 1984. *Morphological and biochemical studies of a naturally occurring enteropathy in the Irish setter dog: a comparison with coeliac disease in man.* Research in Veterinary Science, 37(3):339-46.

Why do dogs eat green grass?

No single answer seems all inclusive. Dogs may eat the grass in the lawns playfully, occasionally, subsequently throwing it up, simply like the taste or eat it for nutritional reasons. Eating grass may be a form of self-treatment for stomach-upset.

8. Feeding habits of wild mammals (additional information to chapter 13)

Wild dogs, also known as hunting dogs, are one of Africa's most successful hunters. With up to 30-players in a pack, they can even take on lions. They go deadly quiet during hunting because any wrong move or a bark can lead their prey to escape. They use ears to act like signaling devices. They can tilt them in different ways to communicate their positions. The pack splits and spaces themselves to form a cordon around the antelope / deer. They gulp down as much food as they can and finish eating quickly. The pack leader feeds the young ones by regurgitating the meat he has eaten.

Chimpanzees chase a troop of monkeys. A 'chaser' chimp would get the monkeys to move. There would be 'blockers' moving into position on the side of the monkey so that he cannot escape. There would be a 'catcher' who comes into play, completing the hunt. Chimpanzees also make a lot of noise on the hunt. It is their way of getting themselves hyped up for the hunt.

Dolphins are generally found in murky waters. They cannot see the fish, so they use their echolocation skills to find the prey. They talk to each other and plan their attack through their whistles and clicks. By swimming in formation they create mini tidal waves that drive shoals of fish out of the water. Lead dolphins stir up a circle of mud that confuses all the fish. The fish think they have been trapped and they start to panic. This results in fish leaping out of water, straight into the dolphins' mouth.

Leopards are social animals. It is not uncommon for many animals to interact and move together with humans. But why do large cats like leopards attack humans? The two most common opinions are: habitat destruction and lack of food. Leopards have always lived close to human settlements and preyed on dogs and goats. Yet human attacks occur only some places or only in some periods.

As for food, a leopard has a home range of about 20 sq.km. and all it needs is about a goat-sized animal per week. This means 52 dogs/goats in that territory in a year (Vidya Athreya, August 16, 2013 The Hindu daily OP-ED, 9). Leopards are territorial with strong social bonds between related females and mother and cubs.

9. Rabies

Rabies is a fatal disease. Rabies is transmitted between specific wild carnivore reservoir hosts, which serve as a source of spill-over infections of other wild carnivores, and infection of domesticated animals and humans.

Trap-neuter-vaccinate-return (TNVR) programmes: Rabies transmission via feral (wild) cats is a public health concern. Domestic cats are an important part of many Americans' lives. But effective control of the 60-100 million feral cats living throughout the country remains problematic. Trap-neuter-vaccinate-return (TNVR) programmes are growing in popularity as alternative to euthanizing feral cats for controlling their populations. However, TNVR has not been shown to reliably reduce feral cat populations because of low implementation rates, inconsistent maintenance and immigration of unsterilized cats into colonies. Roebling et al. (2013) suggested responsible pet ownership, universal rabies vaccination of pets and removal of stray animals need to be complemented because they are integral components to control rabies and other diseases.

It is reported that rabies prevention and control efforts have been successful in reducing or eliminating virus circulation in the United States through vaccination of specific reservoir populations. It is claimed that canine rabies virus variant had been eliminated from the United States and many other countries (Lankau et al., 2013). However, increased international travel and trade can pose risks for rapid, long-distance movements of ill or infected persons or animals. Such travel and trade can result in human exposures to rabies virus.

In the present day of global travel, a proactive coordination among international public health and travel industry partners is warranted to protect human lives and to prevent the movement of viral variants among the host populations (Lankau et al., 2013).

Lankau, E.W., N.J. Cohen, E.S. Jentes, L.E. Adams, T.R. Bell, J.D. Blanton, D. Buttke, G.G. Galland, A.M. Maxted, D.M. Tack, S.H. Waterman, C.E. Rupprecht and N. Marano 2013. Prevention and control of rabies in an age of global travel: A review of travel- and trade-associated rabies events - United States, 1986-2012. Zoonoses and Public Health; this article is a U.S. Government work and is in the public domain in the USA.

Roebling, A.D., D. Johnson, J.D. Blanton, M. Levin, D. Slate, G. Fenwick and C.E. Rupprecht (2013) Rabies prevention and management of cats in the context of trap-neuter-vaccinate-release programmes. Zoonoses and Public Health

10. Avian atherosclerosis (additional information to chapter 19)

Avian atherosclerosis is a common disease affecting most species of birds. Atherosclerotic lesions are prevalent in companion psittacine species. Parrots account for much of the veterinary scientific information on avian atherosclerosis, but the lesions have been described in virtually all avian orders. Suggested risk factors that may promote the development of atherosclerosis include age, gender, species, increased plasma total cholesterol and triglyceride levels, high-energy and high-fat diet, physical inactivity, thyroid disease and coinfection with *Chlamydophila psittaci* (Beaufrere, 2013).

A higher prevalence or severity of atherosclerotic lesions was frequently reported in older birds. Beaufrere et al. (2013) confirmed that female gender and age are important risk factors for atherosclerotic diseases. It is interesting to note that psittacine birds exhibit a reversed sex effect from mammals in which males experience higher prevalence of atherosclerosis. It is reported that in reproductively active females, estrogens induce an increase in plasma total cholesterol and triglyceride levels and hepatic synthesis of 2 specific lipoproteins that target the development of oocyte and are protected against the normal action of plasma lipoprotein lipase (Alvarenga et al., 2011). Thus the increased plasma cholesterol, VLDL, VLDL remnants, and nonhigh-density lipoprotein (HDL) cholesterol levels promote atherogenesis, providing a plausible explanation for the enhanced predisposition found in female psittacine birds.

It was demonstrated that African grey parrots, Amazon parrots, and cockatiels (*Nymphicus hollandicus*) appeared to be atherosclerosis prone (plasma cholesterol level 421 mg/dl), whereas cockatoos (Cacatua spp.) and macaws (Ara spp.) were determined to be somewhat atherosclerosis resistant (plasma cholesterol level 223 mg/dL). It appears that some Psittacine species have evolved different dietary habits in captivity, and accordingly some species may be better equipped to metabolize dietary lipids than others. Experimental diet-induced atherosclerosis was associated with increased plasma total cholesterol level in budgerigars (*Melopsittacus undulatus*) and quaker parrots (*Myiopsitta monachus*) also.

Prevention: Lifestyle changes that could be implemented for companion avian species include increasing physical activity by providing more opportunities for locomotion and foraging behaviours and decreasing the stress level in their captive environment. Limiting dietary excess and obesity also seem to be a reasonable strategy, but species-specific dietary needs should be considered.

Beaufrere, H. (2013) *Avian atherosclerosis*: Parrots and beyond. Journal of Exotic Pet Medicine 22: 336-347.

Beaufrère, *H., Ammersbach, M., Reavill, D., et al.* (2013) Prevalence and risk factors in psittacine athersoclerosis: a multicenter case-control study. J Am Vet Med Assoc 242:1696-1704.

Alvarenga, *R.R., Zangeronimo, M. G., Pereira, L.J., et al.* (2011) Lipoprotein metabolism in poultry. World Poult Sci J 67: 431-440.

11. Canine Hereditary Copper-associated Hepatitis

Copper is an essential dietary nutrient with important functions in many cellular processes. However, in excessive amounts, copper can be toxic due to its potential to facilitate the formation of reactive oxygen species. Several dog breeds have a genetic susceptibility for hepatic copper accumulation. Such breeds include Doberman. Labrador retriever, the Bedlington terrier, West Highland White terrier and the Skye terrier. Canine hereditary copper-associated hepatitis is characterized by gradual hepatic copper accumulation eventually leading to liver cirrhosis. The hepatic copper accumulation may range from about 800 rag up to 5000 mg/kg liver on dry-weight basis. The normal hepatic copper concentrations are less than 400 mg/kg dry weight of the liver.

Therapy is aimed at creating a negative copper balance by promoting urinary copper excretion with metal chelators such as D-penicillamine, the one most commonly used. However, D-penicillamine often causes gastrointestinal side effects including anorexia and vomiting and lethargy, and life-long continuous therapy may lead to a deficiency of copper and zinc.

Fieten et al. (2014) investigated the effect of a low-copper, high-zinc diet as an alternative to continuous D-penicillamine treatment for the long-term management of canine copper-associated hepatitis. Sixteen affected Labrador retrievers (mean age, 6.8±1.4 years; body weight, 33.3±4.5 kg) were followed for a period of 19.1 months (range, 5.9–39 months) after being effectively treated with D-penicillamine (20mg/kg/day for a period of 10.9±4.2 months). The dogs were maintained on a diet containing 1.3 ± 0.3 mg copper/1000 kcal (5.11 mg/DMB) and 64.3 ± 5.9 mg zinc/1000 kcal (243.34 mg/DMB). The diet was a commercially available one with the lowest copper and highest zinc concentration. Copper in the diet came from the raw materials and zinc sulphate was added in a premix. The diet had 8.1% moisture, 17.8% protein, 16.4% fat, 4.5% ash, 50.7% NFE and 2.5% crude fibre with ME of 3.79 Mcal/kg. Liver biopsies were taken every 6 months for histological evaluation and copper determination. Plasma alanine aminotransferase (ALT) and alkaline phosphatase, as well as serum albumin were determined.

Dietary treatment alone was sufficient to maintain hepatic copper concentration below 800 mg/kg dry weight of liver in 12 dogs during the study period. Four dogs needed re-treatment with D-penicillamine. ALT activity and albumin concentration were not associated with hepatic copper concentration, but showed a significant association with the stage and grade of hepatitis respectively. A low-copper, high-zinc diet can be a valuable alternative to continuous D-penicillamine administration for long-term management of dogs with copper-associated hepatitis. The copper re-accumulation rate of an individual dog should be considered in the design of a long-term management protocol and in determining rebiopsy intervals. Factors that could influence the re-accumulation rate of copper such as copper uptake via drinking water and genetic variation between dogs also need to be kept in mind.

Fieten, *R. Biourge, V.C., Watson, A.L., Leegwater, P.A.J., Van den Ingh, T.S.G.A.M and Rothuizen*, J., 2014. Nutritional management of inherited copper-associated hepatitis in the Labrador retriever. The Veterinary Journal, http://dx.doi.org/10.1016/j.tvjl.2013.12.017.

Index